More of
Mould's Medical Anecdotes

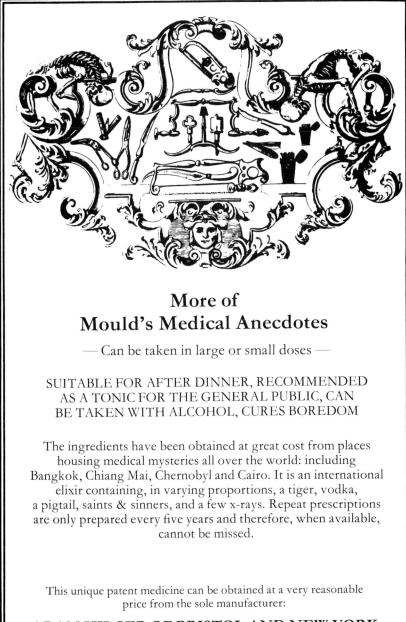

More of
Mould's Medical Anecdotes

— Can be taken in large or small doses —

SUITABLE FOR AFTER DINNER, RECOMMENDED
AS A TONIC FOR THE GENERAL PUBLIC, CAN
BE TAKEN WITH ALCOHOL, CURES BOREDOM

The ingredients have been obtained at great cost from places
housing medical mysteries all over the world: including
Bangkok, Chiang Mai, Chernobyl and Cairo. It is an international
elixir containing, in varying proportions, a tiger, vodka,
a pigtail, saints & sinners, and a few x-rays. Repeat prescriptions
are only prepared every five years and therefore, when available,
cannot be missed.

This unique patent medicine can be obtained at a very reasonable
price from the sole manufacturer:

ADAM HILGER OF BRISTOL AND NEW YORK

or from any respectable bookshop.

British Library Cataloguing in Publication Data

Mould, R. F. (Richard Francis) *1939–*
    More of Mould's medical anecdotes.
    1. Medicine. Humour
    I. Title
    610′.20

ISBN 0-85274-119-7

US Library of Congress Cataloging-in-Publication Data

Mould, Richard F. (Richard Francis)
    More of Mould's medical anecdotes/Richard F. Mould.
    269p. 24cm.
    Includes index.
    ISBN 0-85274-119-7
    1. Medicine—History—Anecdotes. I. Title.   II. Title: Medical
anecdotes.
R705.M69   1989
610′.207—dc20   89-34236
                                                                      CIP

Published under the Adam Hilger imprint by IOP Publishing Ltd
Techno House, Redcliffe Way, Bristol BS1 6NX, England
335 East 45th Street, New York, NY 10017-3483, USA

Typeset by BC Typesetting, Exeter
Printed in Great Britain by J W Arrowsmith Ltd, Bristol

For MAUREEN

Contents

Preface to *More of Mould's Medical Anecdotes*   xiii
Preface to *Mould's Medical Anecdotes*   xv

Nurse and Patient in the Fourteenth Century   1
The Red Cross, 1870   1
Murder by Digits   4
Qualities Needed by a Roman Surgeon, AD 30   4
Voltaire on Physicians   5
The Original Siamese Twins, Chang–Eng Bunker, 1811–74   5
Gorky Park and Gerasimov   9
King Philip of Macedon and the Manchester Mummies   14
Descartes and the Mind   24
The Irish Giant, the Sicilian Dwarf and the American Giant   24
The Wax Museum of Florence University   27
Martin Luther on Medicine, Mathematics and Theology   31
A Plea for the Pigtail   31
Spanish Proverb   32
The Two-headed Nightingale   33
Fire Damage   33
Barnum's Prize Ladies   34
Anecdote on Dr Cunningham   34
The Biddenden Maids   35
Trusses for Ruptures, 1734   36
Hippocratic Hoax   37
Anecdote of George James Guthrie, FRS, Army Surgeon
    to Wellington   37
Pliny on Doctors   39
Why Choose Anaesthetics or Dermatology?   40
Excuses, Excuses!   40
Surgeon's Hazards, Babylon, 1000 BC   41
Anecdote of Dr Gilmore and Dr Graham   41
God and the Doctor   42
Australian Medicine Man with Magic Healing Crystal   42
Physician's Fees in St Louis, 1829   43
Confucius on Medicine   44
An Opinion on Quacks, 1714   44
Cigars to Cure Bronchitis   45
Take a Wine-Moistened Topaz   45
Toothache in the Third Century AD?   49
Oscar Wilde's Dying Words   49
Napoleon on Doctors   50
Medical Ants   50

Pour the Medicine over the Patient's Head   50
Remarkable Prevention of Poaching   51
Gravestone Inscription in America's Rural South   51
'Sorry Sir, But what your Wife wants is not Available on
    Prescription'   52
An Experiment with Rats   52
'In my Spare Time I Shoe Horses'   53
Saint Who's?   53
Caesarean Section by the Patient Herself   58
John Shaw Billings on Statistics   59
Somerset Maugham on Training   59
Childbirth in Sicily   60
Pompeian Surgery and Surgical Instruments   60
Cure for a Babylonian Hangover   68
The Carbolic Smoke Ball   69
Lott's Lung Pills   70
Removal of Stones from the Head   70
A Yorkshire Water Doctor   71
Eleven Blue Men   73
Old Dog, New Tricks   81
A Barber Surgeon Operating in his Office   82
The Indian Manner of Blood-letting   83
Breathing a Vein   84
Rejects   84
Setting Limbs   85
Physician's Tombstone   86
French Proverb   86
Consultation with a Thirteenth-century Arab Physician   87
The Earliest Recorded Clinical Trial   88
Malingering   88
Milk Transfusion   97
Cow Pearl Jam   98
Gin Mania in London   99
Nicholas Copernicus and the Inception of Bread-buttering   102
Irish Proverb   105
Medicinal Uses of Wine   106
Onion Incantation to Exorcise Sickness   106
The Oyster's Consolation   107
Biology Exam Howlers   107
Illustrations from a Twelfth-century Medical Treatise   108
Anecdote of an Australian Professor of Physiology   111
Anecdote of a Roman Medical School, AD 80   112
Anecdote of Nansen   112

Fission of Sir Arthur Conan Doyle into Sherlock Holmes and
    Doctor Watson   113
Zip Answer to Stomach Problem   114
Prisoner Surprises the Police Taking Him to Jail   114
$10 000 Radium used to Cure Sing Sing Convict   115
The Medico-legal Significance of X-rays in the First Year
    after their Discovery   116
The Duc de Richelieu on Handwriting   123
Lord Palmerston's Last Words   123
Radiation Protection in 1910   124
A Specialist   124
Persian Anatomy   125
Philosophy   125
Varicose Veins in Ancient Greece   126
An Adult   126
George Washington's Medical Supplies   127
Derbes's Law   127
The Buck-Passing Machine   128
Seeking Health in Babylon   130
The Pigtail of Li-Fang-Fu   130
Camel Ambulance in Afghanistan   133
Koko for the Hair   134
It's not What you Write—Its the Way that you Write it   135
Is Graphology Accurate? Ask Lord Nelson and the Duke of
    Wellington   139
Finger Reckoning in the Middle Ages   147
Metoposcopy: Observation of the Forehead   148
Charms Against Teething   152
Charm Against Nightmares   153
Rabbit Fights Back   153
Charm Against Rheumatism   154
Suicide   155
Anointing   156
Leonardo's Last Supper   157
The Royal Wedding   159
Treatment of Political Prisoners under a Liberal Government   160
How Diet Changes your Personality   160
Medical English   161
When the Bull Beats the Matador   164
The Many Pains of Snoring   165
A Student's Criminals   165
An Old-time Apothecary   166
The Aetiology and Treatment of Childhood   167
An Italian Quack   173

Anecdote of Field-Marshall Lord Montgomery   174
A Scene of Mesmeric Therapy   174
Samuel Butler's Description of the Human Body   176
Anecdote of Sir Clement Price Thomas   176
Lettsom's Moral and Physical Thermometer   177
Impromptu Speech   178
Anecdote of Virchow and Bismarck   178
The Dinner-plate Twins   178
Advertisement for a Surgeon–Dentist   179
Persian Wisdom   179
The Pestäule in Vienna   179
Miracylous Medical Properties of Russian Vodka   180
Abortions in Greece, January 1987   182
Eyewitness Account of the First Physician at the Scene of the
    Chernobyl Accident, 1986   183
Medical Papyri from Egypt   185
Most-sought-after Plant   187
Manioc is a Root of Good and Evil for the Third World   187
Charlatan Extracting Teeth   190
His First Operation: A Short Story by Sir Arthur Conan Doyle   190
Mr Chamberlen's Secret   196
First Orbiting Space Mausoleum Okayed   201
Man Became Violent after Eating Crisps   201
Anatomical Rhyming Slang   202
The Death of John Partridge in 1708   203
Anecdote of The Earl of Shrewsbury and a Mouse   204
Florence Nightingale and the Crimean War Hospitals, 1854–6   205
A Dropped Catch—The Case of the Bouncing Baby   212
The Mystery of Byron's Corpse   214
Bathtub Elixir puts Estonian behind Bars   219
Capgras Syndrome   220
French X-ray Finds a Screw Loose   220
Self-inflicted Frontal Lobotomy   220
Almost-failed EEC Contraception   221
Premature Burial   222
Yellow Fever Experiment in Cuba   224
Vaccination   224
A Deaf Australian Magistrate   225
Sir Anthony Oyster   226
The Birth of Anaesthesia   228
Florence Nightingale as Medical Statistician, 1859–61   233
Plato on Hiccoughing   242
The Cannon Effect   242
Medicine in Ancient Egypt   243

Anecdote of Aesclepiades of Prusa   247
The First Whole-body X-ray   248
Meo Hill Tribe Herb Doctor in Northern Thailand   249
Anatomical Comparisons by Rabelais   251
Jail Fever in Newgate   251
Diderot on Doctors   253
John Hunter on Operations   253
On Alcoholism   253
Witch from Brittany   254
Moscow Weddings   254
On Filling in Life Insurance Forms   255
Saint Pantaleon   256
On How to Start a Speech in the Apothecaries Hall   256
On Getting Matters into Perspective   257
Gin and Tonic   257
A Moralistic Story about Two Peasants, a Bird and a Cow   257
International Definitions of Heaven and Hell   258
The Frog   258
Sales Opportunities   259
Bulgarian Proverb   259
Irish Proverb   259
A Medical Demon from Angkor Wat   260
Confusion   260

Index   263

Preface to More of Mould's Medical Anecdotes

With my publishers now asking for a second volume of *Anecdotes*, I obviously got the recipe correct in the first volume with its ingredients of quacks, skeletons, x-rays, witch doctors, saints and foreign bodies of various descriptions. A repeat prescription is therefore offered for those who were kind enough, or foolhardy enough, to part with real money on the promise of a few laughs. This collection has, to some extent, been easier to assemble, since many of my friends are now aware that I am an anecdotal squirrel. In consequence, material has been arriving in a steady stream from many countries. I would hasten, though, to apologise to some contributors for the exclusion of their favourite material, because I have felt it paramount to observe a certain amount of decorum with this anthology—most of the time! As before, parts have been gathered whilst I have been abroad on non-trivial matters for WHO, IAEA and other bodies, and consequently the reader will find in these pages mention of events either experienced first hand (such as the case of the Tiger's Penis near the Golden Triangle) or merely reported in local newspapers and books in Cairo, Manila, Bangkok, Chernobyl and Chiang Mai. The spectrum of contents includes, as before, the historical, the unusual, the unexpected, the humorous and the mysterious; from sources such as medical journals, advertisements, comic monologues and newspapers. In addition, I have been able to incorporate material proffered during interviews when the first volume of *Anecdotes* was published. In particular, I must mention Monica O'Hara, who interviewed me for the *Liverpool Echo* and who turned out to be an expert graphologist as well as a journalist. We collaborated with my friend the late Harold Winter to produce the results of the graphology 'blind' trial of Wellington and Nelson. Illustrations again loom large and I am most grateful to the various picture libraries such as those of the Wellcome Library for the History of Medicine and the Mansell Collection. I hope, therefore, that there will be something for everybody in this volume and that it will raise a laugh or two when readers have a few minutes to relax from the daily grind.

Richard F Mould
London, February 1989

Preface to Mould's Medical Anecdotes

I first became attracted to the idea of producing a book of anecdotes during my schooldays some 30 years ago. Imagine my surprise when I later found an 1866 book of anecdotes compiled by one of my ancestors, another Richard Mould (1806–1871), four generations earlier. This book was entitled *Literary Pearls Strung at Random: Historical and Biographical Anecdotes, Aphorisms, Wit and Humour in Prose and Verse.* We obviously share a sense of humour as he had published one epitaph that I had also thought of choosing! This concerns Frederick, Prince of Wales, father of King George III:

> Here lies Fred,
> Gone down among the dead.
> Had it been his Father
> We had much rather;
> Had it been his Mother
> Better than any other;
> Had it been his sister,
> Few would have missed her;
> Had it been the whole generation,
> Ten times better for the nation;
> But since it is only Fred,
> There is nothing more to be said.

However, the impetus to compile this current collection was not so much a wish to follow in family footsteps, but more a response to comments from students on a collection of illustrations used in lectures to keep the audience awake. When in reply to a request for questions I more than once received comments such as 'please tell us some more anecdotes' or 'have you written a book of anecdotes?', a compilation began to seem like a good idea, and gathering these articles together provided light relief while writing books of a more serious nature.

The resultant medical recipe, described on the jacket as a quack medicine, is offered to all those who enjoy reading books of 'snippets' and viewing interesting and unusual illustrations. Particular emphasis has been placed on photographs and the contents cover a spectrum of the historical, the unusual, the unexpected, the humorous and the mysterious. Medical anecdotes have been extracted from many sources including newspaper cuttings, epitaphs, quotations, medical journals, advertisements, comic monologues and case histories, and the subject matter ranges from evolution through animals, politicians, punk rockers and royalty to mummification and death, from medical schools to surgeons, from quacks and witch doctors to saints and from lead poisoning to radioactivity. The compilation also has an international flavour including articles relating to places as far apart as Egypt and Colombia, Russia and the Philippines, and Thailand and Ireland, but asking overseas friends for their favourite medical anecdote did not always provide a publishable reply!

Items have been selected from many medical journals including *British Medical Journal, The Lancet, New England Journal of Medicine* and *Journal of the American Medical Association.* The Wellcome Library for the History of Medicine Provided several of the illustrations and there are also reproductions from the Tate and National Portrait Galleries in London and the Tretyakov Gallery and the Kremlin Faceted Chamber in Moscow. Hopefully, there is something for everyone, particularly those interested in medicine.

Richard F Mould
London, August 1983

Nurse and Patient in the Fourteenth Century

Nurse bathing a patient. Fourteenth century manuscript illustration from a collection in the Royal Palace Library, Lisbon, Portugal.

(Courtesy Wellcome Institute Library, London.)

The Red Cross, 1870

The *Graphic* was a nineteenth century popular magazine, somewhat similar to the *London Illustrated News*, and from time to time carried various illustrations of a medical or nursing nature, such as that of the Red Cross Nurse in 1870, which was by a Mr H Weigall, and was 'put on exhibition for the benefit of the Distressed French Peasantry'. The recent war referred to by the *Graphic* was the Franco–Prussian War which the French lost, and after which Emperor Napoleon III was exiled and died in England. The second illustration is from a later edition of the *Graphic* (September 1876) and is entitled *The Red Cross Quarters in the Field*.

1

The sketch represents an English lady, one of the numerous band of the 'Red Cross' sisterhood, who, during the recent campaigns, have devoted themselves to ministering to the sufferings of the sick and wounded victims of war. Many a refined and delicately nurtured woman has left the luxuries and comforts of her peaceful English home—a voluntary exile, following in the footsteps of a foreign army,

(Courtesy Mansell Collection.)

spending the long sultry days of summer, and the cold dreary nights of winter, in the wards of an army ambulance, often beyond the reach even of letters or news from her native home. Bright and graceful, and withal calm and simple, as the fair subject of our sketch, these true gentlewomen of England have soothed the dying agony, or cheered the weary hours of slow convalescence of many a humble hero. No scenes have been too trying, no work too hard, no services too menial for these devoted women. Wherever the Red Cross Banner has waved, they have been found, women of whom England may well be proud, women of whom doctors and patients speak with equal enthusiasm; gentle, obedient, tender to the sick, with neither theories nor crotchets to work out, simply doing their duty under direction with loving patience and faithfulness. Our sketch depicts a room in one of the many stately old French chateaux, but a few short months ago the home of a prosperous family, the scene of festive gatherings, now the refuge of pain and suffering. The lofty 'salons' converted into hospital wards; camp bedsteads and the rough appliances of a field ambulance replacing the luxurious canopies and inlaid cabinets. The delicately furnished boudoir and 'Chambre de Madame' converted into store rooms, heaps of coarse woollen clothing and piles of bandages filling the wardrobes where gorgeous robes were wont to hang. On the shelves the varied appliances of a fashionable lady's toilet ruthlessly cleared away to make room for neatly-arranged stores of medical comforts and necessaries. The young Englishwoman has evidently with her own hands been opening one of the large well-packed bales, sent by her generous countrywomen. She is now carrying a bundle of bandages into the adjoining ward, where the surgeon is doubtless waiting for her gentle aid to bind up the shattered limb of a patient sufferer, who a few hours ago was marching into battle in all the pride of his youth and strength, now laid low on a bed of pain, grateful for the soothing sympathy and tender care of the English Infirmière. To him she seems a ministering angel, throwing a ray of light upon his sufferings, recalling to him in his hour of agony the fair and loving bride, whose soft-toned voice he longs, with all the longing of a dying exile, once more to hear.

REFERENCE

The *Graphic* 'English Infirmière in a French chateau' 14 January 1871 p. 34

3

Murder by Digits

Swedish authorities have revealed that a computer has 'killed' thousands of citizens. It will take hundreds of hours and cost several million pounds to resurrect the slain Swedes, from Boraas county. The accident happened when a computer operator innocently keyed a request to the county's computer to update its records, and take account of recent deaths.

Unfortunately registers of people in Sweden are based on a six-digit number and a four-digit number, each linked by a hyphen. In defence of its mass murder, the computer only did what it was instructed to do. It interpreted the hyphen as a minus, subtracted the second number from the first, and was left with an unintelligible figure. The computer rejected these figures as obsolete and erased the records from its memory.

The records, and lives, of all these Swedes are now being reinstated manually.

REFERENCE

New Scientist 16 August 1984

Qualities Needed by a Roman Surgeon, 30 AD

The following blueprint for a surgeon was given by Cornelius Celus whose eight volumes 'On Medicine' (*De Medicina*) were written about the year 30 AD in ancient Rome.

A surgeon must be youthful, or at any rate nearer youth than old age. He must have a strong, steady hand, which never trembles, and be no less ready to use the left hand than the right; his eyesight must be sharp and clear, his spirit undaunted. He must be compassionate, so that he wishes to cure the patient in his care, but not to the extent that he is moved by his cries either to go faster than is desirable or to cut less than is necessary; he must do everything just as if the cries of the patient cause him no emotion.

4

Voltaire on Physicians

A physician is a man who pours drugs of which he knows a little into a body of which he knows less.

The Original Siamese Twins, Chang–Eng Bunker, 1811–74

Eng and Chang were born in Siam about May 1811. Their father was of Chinese extraction and had gone to Siam and there married a woman whose father was also a Chinaman. Hence, for the most part, they were of Chinese blood, which probably accounted for their dark colour and Chinese features. Their mother was about 35 years old at the time of their birth and had borne four female children prior to Chang and Eng. She afterwards had twins several times, having eventually 14 children in all. She gave no history of special significance of the pregnancy, although she averred that the head of one and the feet of the other were born at the same time. The twins were both feeble at birth, and Eng continued to be delicate, while Chang thrived. It was only with difficulty that their lives were saved, as Chowpahyi, the reigning king, had a superstition that such freaks of nature always presaged evil to the country.

They were really discovered by Robert Hunter, a British merchant in Bangkok, who in 1824 saw them boating and stripped to the waist. He prevailed on the parents and King Chowpahyi to allow them to go away for exhibition, and they were first taken out of the country by a certain Captain Coffin. The first scientific description of them was given by a Professor Warren who examined them at Harvard University in 1829. At that time Eng was 5′ 2″ and Chang 5′ 1½″ in height. They presented all the characteristics of Chinamen and wore long black pigtails coiled three times about their heads.

After an eight-week tour of the eastern United States they went to London, but a tour of France was forbidden since the French considered that they would possibly cause the production of *monsters* by maternal impressions in pregnant women. After their tour of 1829 they returned to the United States and settled down as farmers in North Carolina, adopting the name of Bunker. When 44 years of age they married two sisters, English women, 26 and 28 years of age respectively. Domestic strife soon compelled them to keep their wives

5

in separate houses, and they visited each wife on alternate weeks. Chang had six children, Eng five, all healthy and strong.

Oil painting by Edward Pingret, 1836. (Courtesy Wellcome Institute Library, London.)

In 1869 they made another trip to Europe, ostensibly to consult the most celebrated surgeons of Great Britain and France on the advisability of being separated. It was stated that a feeling of antagonistic hatred after a quarrel prompted them to seek surgical separation but the real cause was most likely to replenish their depleted finances.

They were never in fact separated, and by 1869 both had diseased arteries, Chang had marked spinal curvature and they were both partially blind in their two anterior eyes. This was possibly due to looking outward and obliquely for so many years. The point of junction was about the sterno-xiphoid angle, and was a band of cartilage extending from sternum to sternum which in 1869 measured 4½″ but during early life was probably not greater than 3″.

The twins died in Januaray 1874, aged 62 years, and at autopsy it was found that there was a hepatic connection through the band to their two livers with slight intercommunication of the blood supply to the livers, but that they had independent peritoneal cavities and intestines.

The term *monster* was used for many years to describe the union of two foetuses and the x-ray picture shows what was termed a *skiagram of a double monster,* published in 1896 in the *Archives of Clinical Skiagraphy, London,* the forerunner of the *Archives of the Roentgen Ray* and the *Journal of the Röntgen Society.* It is therefore the world's first published radiograph of Siamese twins.

SKIAGRAM OF A DOUBLE MONSTER

(By J. LYNN THOMAS, F.R.C.S., Cardiff.)

Not all foetuses are joined by a band of cartilage, as Chang–Eng, and the possible variants include:

(*a*) union of two distinct foetuses by a bony junction of the heads;

(*b*) union of two distinct foetuses in which one or more parts are eliminated by the junction;

(*c*) fusion of two foetuses by a bony union at the pelvis;

(*d*) fusion of two foetuses below the umbilicus into a common lower extremity.

In addition, there are also instances of *bicephalic monsters* which are single foetuses with the exception of having two heads and two necks and *parasitic monsters* which consist of one perfect body complete in every respect, but from the neighbourhood of whose umbilicus depends some important portion of a second body.

These unfortunate specimens of humanity were invariably placed on show, as the advertisement of August 1838 illustrates.

(Courtesy Wellcome Institute Library, London.)

REFERENCES

Gould G M and Pyle W L 1900 *Anomalies and Curiosities of Medicine* (Philadelphia: Saunders)

Rogers A 'Siamese twins' *Hospital Doctor* 12 March 1981

Gorky Park and Gerasimov

In the well known Russian-set thriller *Gorky Park*,[1] which was also turned into a successful film of drama, intrigue and smuggling, three bodies are found in Moscow's Gorky Park with the soft tissues of their faces completely ripped away to avoid identification. Later, they were reconstructed by a Russian professor as an integral part of the plot.

Most readers and film viewers probably assume that this professor was a figment of the author's imagination, but in actual fact he really did exist and was Professor Mikhail Gerasimov, who until his death in 1970 was the Director of the Laboratory of Plastic Reconstruction at the Ethnographical Institute of the USSR in Moscow. His work was confined mostly to the faces of the paleolithic man and historical figures such as Ivan the Terrible,[3] but he did work on some one hundred forensic reconstructions and some of his achievements are described below from the book by Smyth.[2] The photographs were taken in Moscow and are published by courtesy of the Novosti Press Agency.

When he died in July 1970, Professor Mikhail Gerasimov was world famous not only in the field of palaeontology—his own discipline—but also in that of forensic medicine, for it was through his efforts that Russia came to the fore in the facial reconstruction branch of criminal science. As far back as 1950 Professor Gerasimov had been instrumental in the setting up of the Laboratory for Plastic Reconstruction, which forms part of the Ethnographical Institute of the USSR Academy of Sciences; since then the laboratory has assisted Russian investigators in the solving of hundreds of crimes.

Gerasimov was born in St Petersburg—later Leningrad—in 1907 and took a precocious interest in archaeology and palaentology. As early as 1920, when he was 13, he had become a part-time student at the University of Irkutsk, in Siberia, attending lectures in archaeology, ethnography, zoology and medicine. He was also fortunate in gaining the patronage of Professor A.D. Grigoriev, holder of the chair of forensic science, who encouraged the youthful Gerasimov in his interest in the morphology of the human skull.

The task which faced Gerasimov was a complex one; firstly, he had to establish some form of set measurement from those parts of the skull which remained more or less constant—where, that is, the flesh lay thinnest on the bone. Then, much more difficult, he had to discover a system of determining the muscular structure of an individual head. As he put it:

The essence of the programme was that not only definite information about the thickness of the soft parts must be found, but also morphological features of the skull which could serve as clues for the reconstruction of the different parts of the face—nose, mouth, eyes and so forth.

Mikhail Gerasimov selecting material for the second issue of his Atlas *which includes portraits of ancient people (Paleolithic and neolithic) who lived in the Soviet Union, (Photography March 1961. Courtesy Novosti Press Agency.)*

Gerasimov spent two years measuring and dissecting the heads of corpses in the medical faculty of the university before attempting a reconstruction. He was disappointed with his first attempt and showed it to no-one. In 1925, however, he produced a portrait based on a contemporary skull which encouraged both him and Professor Grigoriev. That year he was appointed scientific technical assistant to the Irkutsk Museum, and was later put in charge of its archaeological section; there he reconstructed fossil heads, while at the same time persevering with his experiments on 'fleshed' heads.

It was not until 1935, 15 years after his first tentative steps had been taken, that an opportunity presented itself to prove to his colleagues that he was not driven by, as he put it, 'mania and fanaticism'. In the medical school he found the skeleton of a Dr Kolesnikov, who had left his body for research. Gerasimov had not known the doctor during his lifetime and had never seen a picture of him; however he was told that Kolesnikov's family had snapshots of him taken just before his death.

Carefully, Gerasimov set to work and produced on the skull the features of a man with a high, narrow forehead, a long nose, deep-set little eyes, a large though receding chin and protruding ears; despite this unprepossessing appearance Gerasimov judged that the muscular structure must have given the man a slightly smiling appearance, which 'lent the whole visage a surprising charm'. When Dr Kolesnikov's mother saw the reconstructed head she was at first shocked then deeply moved; her collection of photographs showed the scientist how accurate he had been, and he presented the mother with the portrait.

The same year, Gerasimov's work received what at first he thought to be a setback. He was handed the skull of a Frenchman, one Loustalot, a famous boxer and fencing master who had taught athletics at Leningrad. Gerasimov constructed a likeness in his usual fashion, and then went to compare it with Loustalot's death mask, which was preserved at the Anatomical Institute in Leningrad. To his profound disappointment, only the forehead and twice-broken nose tallied with the death mask.

> The whole of the lower part of the face was different and I would say even alien—strange. The face was noticably broader, as though bloated. The blurred eyes projecting from their orbits and the swollen mouth with thick, shapeless lips were quite unlike those of the face modelled by me.

To Gerasimov's relief there was an explanation. Loustalot had dropped dead in the street, and some time passed before the body was identified. By the time his identity was established, decomposition was fairly advanced, though a death mask had been taken from the decaying features nonetheless. When the portrait was compared with pictures of Loustalot in life, it was found to be as accurate as Dr Kolesnikov's had been.

Professor Grigoriev was delighted with his pupil's progress, and in 1939 gave him his first criminological task. In a wood outside Leningrad numerous bones had been found, scattered over a fairly wide area. They bore the marks of animal teeth, and it was assumed that they were the remains of someone who had been attacked and killed by wolves. However the skull and lower jaw told a different tale; when Gerasimov examined it he found the marks of what he considered to be a small hunting hatchet, along with a fracture which had been made by a blunt instrument. Adhering to the crown were a number of reddish-blonde hairs, which had been cut short some days before death.

The incomplete bone formation, the open sutures on the skull vault, the absence of wisdom teeth and the light wear on the adult teeth suggested to Gerasimov that the individual had been between twelve and thirteen years old. Sexing the head was difficult in view of the age, but the strongly developed supraorbital region and the large mastoid processes among other features seemed to point to the victim having been a boy.

After carefully refitting the lower jaw into place, Gerasimov modelled the most important masticatory muscles—these determine the whole shape of the face. Little by little he remodelled the head taking

11

into account such factors as the individual pecularities in the relief of the skull, the nasal bones and the chin eminence. The result was a snub-nosed, chubby-cheeked boy with a high forehead, a thick upper lip and slightly projecting ears. Short, red-blonde hair was finally added.

Meanwhile, the police had been searching their missing persons files for likely identities. Among them was a folio on a boy who, his parents believed, had run off to Leningrad six months previously. So as not to alarm them unduly, photographs of the reconstructed head were mixed in with 30 photographs of boys of similar age. The father immediately recognized the reconstruction as his son, and when the photograph was circulated the boy's movements were traced. As a result his attacker was caught and brought to trial: 'the first attempt to use a skull reconstruction in a criminal case was thus brilliantly successful' wrote Gerasimov, with justifiable pride.

Throughout the 1940s Gerasimov's fame grew in legal circles, and triumph followed triumph as his techniques became less empirical and more exact. Soon he was training students and by 1950 he had sufficient skilled pupils to establish his Laboratory for Plastic Reconstruction. With each case, he learned a little more about the morphology of the human face, but perhaps one final example suffices best to show how far he had come since his first tentative efforts in 1925.

Shortly after the setting up of the Laboratory, Gerasimov was called upon to reconstruct the face of an elderly woman whose skeleton had been found in a hut in remote woodlands. About a year earlier, the wife of a forester had disappeared in odd circumstances; her husband had said that she had set off to visit their son in a neighbouring town, but neither arrived at her destination nor returned home.

When Gerasimov examined the skull he found it severely damaged; the lower jaw was missing and only three molars in the upper jaw remained intact, the broken roots of the others remaining embedded in the skull. The roof of the mouth was peppered with small round holes, and in the base of the skull Gerasimov found several lead pellets. From this evidence he easily came to the conclusion that the woman had been killed by a shotgun blast from very close quarters.

Careful measuring of the remaining skull and comparison with other measurements in his files gave Gerasimov an idea of the shape of the missing lower jaw, and he was able to build this up in plaster, along with reconstructed teeth. His finished head resembled the missing wife so accurately that the forester confessed.

He had set out to drive his wife to their son's home in his horse-drawn wagon, but on the road there had been an argument. The forester had jumped from the wagon in a fury, telling his wife to drive herself; because the woods were haunted by wolves he had dragged down his double-barrelled shotgun from the back of the wagon, but in his irritation he mishandled the gun, and both barrels went off, one tearing away the bottom of his wife's face, the other hitting her in the chest. In a panic he had hidden the body. After hearing his story and reconstructing the crime, police were convinced that he was telling the truth and he thus avoided a capital charge.

Gerasimov reconstructing the head of the Tadjik poet Rudaki, who died in the tenth century. Basing his work on a detailed study of the way in which the muscles and cartilage of the face and neck were developed, he was able to build fleshed heads that corresponded closely to the living figure. He applied this technique both to heads of which portraits survived and to the heads of prehistoric and historic men and women. (Courtesy Novosti Press Agency.)

Despite Professor Gerasimov's success, Western criminologists have so far seldom followed the lead he has given—a fact which puzzles the more progressive among them. In the course of the past twenty years or so, the widespread use of such techniques as 'identikit' and 'photo-fit' to reconstruct the faces of wanted or missing persons from their description have made the processes familiar to the general public. They have also been used in the identification of corpses and there is little question that their effectiveness would be increased enormously were they to be taken in conjunction with the Gerasimov system.

What is perhaps more extraordinary is the fact that Western forensic odontology has lagged behind the work done by the Russians; Gerasimov attached great importance to teeth as a factor in criminal identification, and in fact the history of dental identification is ancient. Agrippina had an enemy killed, and satisfied herself that the right man had died by examining his teeth. In more recent years the victims of two disastrous fires—at the Vienna Opera House in 1878 and the Paris Charité in 1897—were identified by their teeth. And yet one of Europe's few experts, Professor Gosta Gustafson, writing in the *Criminologist* magazine in 1969, had to report that only three major forensic odontology departments existed in any of the world's dental schools—one in Norway, one in Denmark and one in Cuba.

REFERENCES
[1] Smith M C 1981 *Gorky Park* (London: Collins)
[2] Smyth F 1980 *Cause of Death* (London: Orbis)
[3] Mould R F 1984 'Ivan the Terrible's Skeleton' *Mould's Medical Anecdotes* (Bristol: Adam Hilger) p. 8

King Philip of Macedon and The Manchester Mummies

Gerasimov is not the only person to attempt facial reconstructions, and the group at Manchester University under the direction of Dr Rosalie David and including the medical artist Richard Neave is famous for their work on ancient Egyptian mummified remains. In addition, Neave and his colleagues have provided a fascinating reconstruction of a skull from a royal grave in Vergina, Macedonia, which they have proved beyond reasonable doubt to be that of King Philip II of Macedon, the father of Alexander the Great. This is their story.

THE TWO BROTHERS

The size and shape of a human head is determined largely by the underlying bone structure, as are the facial features, the skull being the matrix upon which the head and face are built. Detailed examination of the skull can generally reveal the age and sex of the individual, and characteristics peculiar to race or ethnic group may also be apparent. The condition of the teeth provides valuable information. The configuration of muscle attachments provides evidence of size and strength, although in the face these are confined mainly to the base of the skull and the lower jaw. It is therefore possible, in principle, to reconstruct the major features of the human head with

14

some degree of accuracy. However, a reconstruction can reveal only the type of face that *may* have existed, the position and general shape of the main features being accurate, but reconstructions of subtle details such as wrinkles and folds being inevitably speculative as there is no factual evidence as to their form or even their existence. Nevertheless, the achievement of the Manchester group is most impressive.

The interest of the Manchester Museum in Egyptology first became apparent to the general public via the press of the day in 1907 when Dr Margaret Murray, Egyptologist to the museum, undertook one of the earliest scientific investigations of Egyptian mummies when she unwrapped and dissected the mummies of the *Two Brothers*, before an invited audience in a large lecture theatre at Manchester University. Her experiment was unique in that she headed an interdisciplinary team whose members were specialists in the fields of anatomy, chemical analysis and the study of textiles. They all contributed knowledge to the detailed examination of these mummies, and the results of their investigations were published in 1910 the book entitled *The Tomb of the Two Brothers*. In the 1970s for the first attempts at facial reconstruction, the skulls of these two brothers were chosen.

The skulls of the two brothers Khnum-Nakht (right) and Nekht-Ankh (left). They were buried together in the rock-tombs of Der-Rifeh and date from the twelfth Dynasty.

Within the coffins of the two brothers were two small statuettes, 15.5 and 25.4 cm high and carved from wood. These represented the

15

deceased as they had been when in full health and so skilfully were they carved that it was decided to make some comparisons of the heads of the statues, which were some 3 cm long, with the life-size reconstructions in the form of clay busts. The head of the statuette of Khnum-Nakht is powerfully built, with full lips and a broad nose and from the hieroglyphics on the coffins it appears that he was the younger of the two, a half-brother to Nekht-Ankh sharing the same mother but with a negro father. He is estimated to have been between 40 and 45 years old at death, and to have suffered from osteo-arthritis which seriously affected his back. After reconstruction, a sketch was made from the clay bust and although the similarity between the drawing and the statuette's head is not striking, it is unmistakable, in spite of the differences in size being so extreme.

The wooden figure of Khnum-Nakht which was found in the coffin.   *The wooden figure of Nekht-Ankh which was found in the coffin.*

The head of the second statuette, Nekht-Ankh, is quite different from that of his half-brother, being more lightly formed and possessing a rather more delicate nose and a smaller mouth and chin. The similarity between statuette and reconstruction was again unmistakable. This elder brother was estimated to have been about 60 years old at death.

16

Sketch of Knhum-Nakht made from the life-size clay model reconstruction.

'1770'—A 13-YEAR-OLD EGYPTIAN GIRL

The skulls of the *Two Brothers* were virtually unbroken, but the third mummy whose face was to be reconstructed by the Manchester group, labelled by them '1770' since no name was known and she was only an anonymous mummy No 1770 in their records, provided more of a problem. The skull had been broken into some 30–40 pieces but, fortunately, the majority of the bones which form the face were largely undamaged, although covered by a thick layer of mud and packing. The mandible was fractured to the left of the midline and both mandibular heads were broken, the vault was totally shattered with many pieces missing. The first stage in the facial reconstruction process was therefore, for 1770, to rebuild the skull in plastic.

The conservation of specimens of such antiquity as Egyptian mummies is of prime importance, and thus before any reconstruction work can be undertaken it is necessary to make accurate casts of a skull. The technique, using plaster of Paris and alginate, is similar to that used for manufacturing plastic face casts for certain radiotherapy patients so that they may be fixed into the correct treatment position before x-rays or gamma rays are delivered from a purpose-built machine such as a linear accelerator (for x-rays) or a cobalt-60 unit (for gamma rays). The reconstruction of the soft tissues on the prepared plaster skull was commenced by first *blocking-in* with soft modelling clay the head, neck and face, allowing the features to develop naturally and it is interesting to note how a skull will start to take on the character of a face at a very early stage.

Skull fragments of 1770 prior to reconstruction. Information provided by the remains of 1770 was somewhat limited at the time of making the reconstruction. Both legs appeared to have been amputated, one above and one below the knee, but whether before or after death was not known. There was evidence to indicate some intestinal infection, and an irregularity in the formation of the bone in the region of the nose suggests the probability of nasal congestion, which may have given rise to a slightly adenoidal appearance.

The muscles of the face are so delicate and fine that they leave very few marks on bones to indicate their origins or insertions. Cartilage forms a large part of the nose, and fat is also an integral part of the soft tissue of the face. As the controlling factor in facial reconstruction was to be soft tissue, there seemed to the Manchester group little point in following anatomical structures too closely. Measurements were made, the thickness of the clay being increased or decreased as necessary until it corresponded to the mean of the maximum and minimum thicknesses for soft tissue of the face at 21 specific points as described by Kollmann and Büchly in 1898[†]. The measurements were taken by passing a thin steel probe through the clay at specific points. A slight variation of this system was adopted for 1770 in that

[†] 'Persistance of the strain and the reconstruction of the physiognomy of the pre-historic skull' *Arch. Anthropol.* **25** 345–59.

pegs cut to the appropriate length were fixed in position on the plaster skull. The clay was built up until it was of the correct thickness. Adjustments were made at the stage when the clay model was completed, which enabled minor ethnic considerations to be highlighted. These involved the eyes, which in ancient Egyptians were more almond shaped, and the tip of the nose. In addition, with 1770, some artistic licence was taken to avoid the somewhat cadaverous look of the *Two Brothers*, bearing in mind that 1770 was an adolescent.

The final reconstruction of 1770 was in many ways very satisfactory to the Manchester group because they were able to give some form of identity to a handful of broken bones, rather than reconstruct from almost perfect skulls, as in the case of the *Two Brothers*. 1770 was therefore taken a stage further than clay bust only. Glass eyes were fitted, eyelashes added, colour given to mouth and skin together with a limited amount of make-up which would almost certainly have been worn by a girl of this age. The hair (reputed to have been obtained from the theatrical props of the television series *Brideshead Revisited*!) was added in the form of a wig, but was only for exhibition purposes and was in no way judged to be part of the scientific reconstruction process. The result is startling and lifelike as can be seen from the photograph.

The final bust of 1770.

1770 contributed one final surprise to her reconstructors in that radiocarbon dating showed that although the bandages around the

19

mummy dated from between AD 105 and AD 405, 1770 was in fact very much older than had been suspected, even though it had been thought that the mummy might have been re-wrapped at some stage. The bones dated from somewhere between 1250 BC and 1600 BC!

ALEXANDER THE GREAT'S FATHER

The *Two Brothers* and *1770* are in no way famous historical figures with a reasonably well documented past. They were just three ordinary Egyptians of their time. There is, however, nothing ordinary about the last case history on reconstruction, one in which a member of the Manchester group was involved, Mr Richard Neave of the Department of Medical Illustration at Manchester University.

In late 1977, Professor Manolis Andronicos of the University of Thessaloniki discovered first two graves and later a third while excavating the Great Tumulus at Vergina in Macedonia: he has himself described the excitement of the discovery, the culmination of a long series of campaigns, on numerous occasions both in lectures around the world and in print. The principal burial was in a barrel-vaulted chamber, with a second burial in an antechamber, a cist tomb at the side contained the remains of a third body. There was little doubt that the burials were royal, not only because of the quality and wealth of the grave-goods—gold and silver, ivory, bronze vessels, armour of all kinds—but also because of the cremated bones in the antechamber and the main tombs were found wrapped in cloth of purple wool and gold thread placed inside magnificent gold *larnakes*, or chests, on each of which was emblazoned a starburst, the emblem of the Macedonian royal house. It confirmed the identification of Vergina with ancient Aigai, the first capital of Macedon and the traditional burial-place of its kings even after the capital was moved to Pella.

It was possible, to say the least, that the occupant of the principal tomb was the father of Alexander the Great, Philip II of Macedon, who was assassinated in 336 BC, and on many grounds he seemed a much more likely candidate than the other names put forward, such as Philip III Arrhidaeus, the mentaly ill half-brother and successor of Alexander who was murdered in 317 BC. However, apart from one name of indirect relevance engraved on a silver strainer found in the main tomb there were no inscriptions, and the dating evidence provided by the metalwork and the black-glazed pottery was inconclusive. Some scholars thought that it sat more comfortably at the end of the fourth century BC; it was also argued that the silver-gilt diadem found in the main tomb was the crown of Macedon adopted after Alexander's campaigns in Persia, and that the Macedonians could only have learnt the technique of constructing a barrel vault during these campaigns.

Andronicos himself felt that Philip II was the most probable occupant, but he was not prepared to commit himself until proof could be found. Although excavations at Vergina are still continuing and further exciting discoveries are still being made, he felt that in view of their importance he should publish a preliminary account— by no means an automatic procedure in Greece. However, this only fuelled the controversy, which seemed unlikely to be settled before the eventual publication of the final report, inevitably still some years off.

The proof that Andronicos needed came from an unexpected quarter, by a series of happy coincidences. Richard Neave, who had been working on reconstruction of the heads of three Egyptian mummies, expressed an interest in working on some Greek skulls.

In 1981 Richard Neave went to Thessaloniki, where, with the ready cooperation of the staff of the Archaeological Museum, he was able to take casts of the bones of the skull. Although the body had been cremated, in general the bones were in remarkably good condition. Nevertheless, the skull was in fragments: the back had been blown out during the cremation, and as one tried to piece the fragments together it was clear that there was some distortion. At this point a two-pronged approach was adopted by showing casts to anatomists and to plastic surgeons.

The discoveries became more and more exciting. First of all it was found that although the heat of the cremation had made the bones shrink by around 10%, it had in general produced very little distortion. In fact detailed study confirmed that the malformation that was causing problems in fitting the pieces together was largely the result of injury and of congenital deformity. This was particularly striking on the mandible and at the right eye-socket, although other anomalies were noted on the upper jaw and the right cheek-bone.

On the mandible the heights of the right condyle, coronoid process and incisura are much greater than those of the left, the right ramus is broader than the left, and there are some other anomalies: in layman's language, the right side of the jaw is higher and more developed than the left. At some stage too the chin and the dental midline have become realigned for reasons that are still unclear to us, so that the natural midline between the central incisors now lies visibly to the right. In short, the left side of the dead man's face was markedly under developed, and the right side over developed, to compensate for this. Yet such is the ability of the human body to make up for such defects that it was probably hardly noticeable to his contemporaries, particularly if he wore the short, thick beard typical of Macedonians before the reign of Alexander. In fact the mandible shows traces of such compensation in additional bone growth at the new centrepoint; on the other hand very few faces are exactly symmetrical anyway.

The plastic surgeons who examined the casts also noted injuries to the right eye-socket: a notch on the upper margin of the right orbit and traces of a healed fracture on the zygomatic bone (the cheek-bone) below it. These they concluded could only have been caused by a missile coming from above. *The eye injury provided the conclusive proof of the identification of the dead man*, and eliminated the possibility that it was Philip III Arrhideaus.

(Left) The reconstructed skull of King Philip II of Macedon showing the line taken by the missile, which injured the right eye. The white parts are casts of the surviving bones and the grey area is the clay in which the bones are set. It also includes the missing areas.

(Right) Wax cast of the reconstructed head of King Philip II. The technique used was similar to that previously described for the Two Brothers and for 1770. It contains hair, beard and skin colouring, shows the scar to the right eye, and a prominent nose. This 'nasal decision' was made since a nose with a prominent bridge was typical of the Macedonian Royal Family, including Alexander the Great.

The published portraits of Philip II of Macedon, the father of Alexander the Great are a gold medallion from Tarsus, now in Paris, made at the time of Caracalla; a marble head in Copenhagen, of

22

Trajanic date but based on an original of a very striking miniature ivory, one of a set found in the tomb at Vergina which must originally have decorated a bier or couch; and a small late Hellenistic marble head in Chicago. All give the impression of a bearded man with a square face having marked brow-ridges, a nose with a pronounced bridge, and an obstinate chin. The most striking feature, however, is that the Copenhagen and Vergina versions show an injury to the right eye, depicted as a nick to the eyebrow with an apparently sightless right eye, rendered on the Chicago marble as a hollow eye-socket.

The Athenian orator Demosthenes, an implacable opponent of Philip, lists the injuries that he was prepared to suffer for the sake of the empire, power, and glory—to have an eye cut out, his collar-bone broken, his hand and leg maimed. The grammarian Didymus Chalcenterus who wrote a commentary on Demosthenes in the first century BC, drawing on various fourth century sources now lost to us, enlarges on this and says quite categorically that 'he had his right eye cut out when he was struck by an arrow while inspecting the siege engines and the protective sheds at the siege of Methone'. This was in 354 BC, eighteen years before his assasination. Didymus' account is confirmed by other ancient authors—and it tallies exactly with the injury we noted on the skull from Vergina.

The proof was provided.

REFERENCES

David A R 1978 *Mysteries of the Mummies* (London: Book Club Associates)
David A R 1979 *Manchester Museum Mummy Project* (Manchester: Manchester University Press)
Marsh B 1984 'Faces from the past' *World Medicine* 21 Jan. 19–21
Neave R A H 1979 'Reconstruction of the heads of three ancient Egyptian mummies *J. Audiovisual Media in Medicine* 2 156–64
Neave R A H 1979 'Mummies waren eens mensen' *Organorama* 4 17–20
Neave R A H, Barson A J and Percy S 1976 'Models for medical teaching' *Medical and Biological Illustration* 26 211–18
Prag J 1984 The flesh on the bones *Popular Archeology* 5 (March) 8–11

ACKNOWLEDGMENT

I am most grateful to Richard Neave for his first-hand story-telling of these most interesting and unusual events. For the section on Philip II, I have drawn closely on the paper by the archeologist John Prag. The illustrations are by courtesy of the Manchester University Department of Medical Illustration, Royal Infirmary, Manchester.

Descartes and the Mind

It is not enough to have a good mind: the main thing is to use it well.

The Irish Giant, The Sicilian Dwarf and the American Giant

The exhibit no visitor to the Hunterian Museum in the Royal College of Surgeons, Lincolns Inn Fields, London, should miss is the glass case containing the skeletons of two giants and one dwarf, together with a giant boot and glove; the death mask, shoes, ring and some wax anatomical impressions of the dwarf.

John Hunter painted by Sir Joshua Reynolds. The feet of the Irish Giant can be seen in the top right-hand corner of the portrait.

John Hunter (1728–93) was the founder of modern scientific surgery, and he investigated, both by dissection and experiment, human and comparative anatomy, and pathology. His museum differed from others in existence during the latter half of the eighteenth century since it was not only a collection of exhibits but also an illustration of his theories—in particular, of the constant adaption in living things of structure to function. Hunter also obviously realised the value of his unique collection and expressed a wish that it should not be sold piecemeal but preserved as an entity.

The American Giant, the Sicilian Dwarf and the Irish Giant, in the Hunterian Museum in the Royal College of Surgeons, London. By kind permission of the President and Council of the Royal College of Surgeons.

25

THE IRISH GIANT

This was Charles Byrne, born in Ireland in 1761 and died in London 1783. When he was exhibited in London he was known as *O'Brian, The Irish Giant* and contemporary newspaper accounts gave his height variously as 8', 8' 2" and 8' 4". These were all exaggerations as the actual height of the skeleton, with due allowance for intravertebral substances, is only 7' 7". There is no verified account of how Hunter came to possess the giant's body, and at the time it was legal to dissect only the bodies of executed criminals and of suicides. The popular version of events is that Hunter told the Irishman 'Giants are usually short lived. Your body has scientific value, so when you die, it should be left to me for dissection'. The terrified giant fled from Hunter, and on later falling ill made his undertaker promise that after death his body would be sunk in a lead-lined coffin off the Thames estuary. Hearing this, some medical students constructed a diving bell, so they could recover the body. However, this was not needed since Hunter bribed the undertakers with £500 to deliver the coffin to his house in Earls Court—where he prepared the skeleton in a large boiler.

THE AMERICAN GIANT

On 17 March 1843, the American, Charles Freeman, appeared on stage in London at the Olympic Theatre with a dwarf named Signor Hervio Nano, in a piece specially written for the pair, entitled *The Son of the Desert and the Demon Changeling*. Ten years later, in 1853, Freeman was serving behind the bar of the Lion and Ball public house at 63 Red Lion Street, Holborn, claiming a height of 7' 6" and a weight of 21 stone. One of his handbills poetically invited the members of the general public to visit him.

> You need not unto Hyde Park go,
> For without imposition
> Smith's Bar Man is, and no mistake
> The true Great Exhibition.
>
> The proudest noble in the land,
> Despite caprice and whim,
> Though looking *down* on all the world,
> Must fain look *up* to him.
>
> His rest can never be disturbed,
> By chanticler in song,
> For though he early goes to bed,
> He sleeps so very *long*.

Though you may boast of many friends,
  Look in and stand a pot,
You'll make a new acquaintanceship,
  The *longest* you have got.

Then come and see the Giant Youth,
  Give Edward Smith a call,
Remember in Red Lion Street,
  The Lion and the Ball.

Freeman's skeleton was not as tall as 7′ 6″ but was only 6′ 8½″. He died in 1854, and in September of that year his bones were purchased for £2 and articulated for display by a Mr Willmost for the sum of £4 12s. 6d.

THE SICILIAN DWARF

With a Sicilian father and an Italian mother, Caroline Crachami (1815–24) was brought to England at the end of the summer of 1823 and exhibited at Oxford, Birmingham, Liverpool and in Bond Street, London. Her parents and four brothers and sisters were all of normal size. Her skeleton is 19.8″ high.

REFERENCES
Silverberg R 1968 'Anatomy of a surgeon' *Reader's Digest* (December)
Allen E 1974 *Guide to the Hunterian Museum* (London: Royal College of Surgeons of England)
Exhibit captions in the Hunterian Museum

The Wax Museum of Florence University

For many years the dissection of corpses for medical teaching in anatomy was dissaproved by church authorities and in most centres the educational material was limited to diagrams. However, in Florence in the eighteenth century the study of anatomy was greatly assisted by the use of wax models, culminating in the work of Clemente Susini (1754–1805) who was famous not only for the amazing number of waxworks he executed during his lifetime, but also for the high standard of his techniques. He was assisted by several first-class anatomists, including Paolo Mascagni (1755–1815) who was a specialist on the lymphatic system and the author of excellent anatomical drawings. There are now over a thousand models on exhibition at *La Specola* (so called, because in 1780 a telescope was placed on top of the building for astronomical observations and this event stirred the public imagination to such an extent that the whole museum—originally called the Royal and Imperial Museum of Physics and Natural History when it first opened in 1775—was called 'la Specola' from specula meaning look-out, observatory). This is the Zoological Museum of Florence University and is to be found in the Via Romana, the old road from Florence to Rome, and is open to the general public on only one half-day per week. The models on display are contained in their original eighteenth-century glass cases and one of the most impressive is a whole life-sized body illustrating the lymphatic system, and known as *the skinned man*. In addition to the work of Susini there are also some models from the seventeenth century, by the abbé Gaetano Giulio Zummo or Zumbo (1665–1701) who worked for several masters such as the Medici in Florence and Louis XIV in Paris. Only a few examples of his work have survived to the present day, and these include an anatomy of a man's head.

The skinned man by Clemente Susini (1754–1805).

Although dissection of corpses for medical purposes was supposed to be banned by the church, a large number of bodies for dissection were nevertheless obtained by the wax modellers of Florence, and according to papers in the State Archives these bodies had to be duly recorded by a doorman in a daily register. The burdensome task of

28

Anatomy of a man's head by Gaetano Zumbo (1656–1701).

transporting these corpses to and from the Santa Maria Nuova Hospital fell to one Giacinto Guidetti, the cleaner who each day made his gruesome rounds with a basket. The Florentine Archives contain many of his pleas, the most pathetic of which might be that dated 29 November 1792 in which he asked for . . .*a waxed hat, a coat and a pair of boots, so that in transporting corpses to and from the Hospital I am protected from the rain and cold, as it is not possible for me to stop anywhere along the way with the basket. . . .* The Archives also tell us that in January 1790 the Grand Duke of Florence approved of dividing the morning into two sessions, the first for the populace and the second for intelligent people of consequence!

The techniques followed by the wax modellers varied according to the size and nature of the piece to be reproduced; the smaller the model, the more delicate the process.

As far as the larger models are concerned, they were copied from the actual limb or corpse dissected expressly by an anatomist for the purpose; drawings from scientific books were of much aid (those of Paolo Mascagni were extremely useful for this purpose). A model in coarse wax or in clay was made and subsequently a plaster mould was made on it. Once the mould was ready, it was rubbed inside with soft soap in order to fill the small pores and to facilitate the subsequent detachment of the model. After this was dried, a first layer of soft wax was spread inside and given the general background colour, yellowish if it was a skin, dark red for the liver, and so on. The thickness of this layer varied according to the size of the piece to be reproduced. When this had been cooled a second layer of wax of about the same thickness was added on the first one, and in the case of a large piece, a third thicker layer was added. It is likely that in the most carefully executed pieces, the first step before these rough layers were poured inside, was to cover the mould with a thin layer of almost fluid wax, applied with a paint-brush, having a colour somewhat deeper or paler than the underlying material, according to the effect which was desired.

For the largest pieces of work like thorax and abdomen with all the viscera, it was necessary to improve the solidity; in this case the cast was left open on the underside and, when the wax layers were cooled, the cavity was filled with tow impregnated with wax. In the case of organs such as the liver, kidneys, lungs and stomach, which appear in the more complex compositions, these were modelled separately, and by being warmed were welded to the common base with wax.

The full-bodied models, both the standing and the lying ones, bear inside an iron frame, accurately shaped in the attitude which the body is expected to show. This iron frame was well wrapped in tow and cloth soaked with wax in order to prevent the finished statue from sliding along it; the remaining cavities were filled in the same way. The whole figure was not cast in one piece; the head, bust, arms and legs were prepared separately and eventually joined together at a later stage.

The striations of the muscle fibres were made on the finished model, then the nerves, lymphatics and blood-vessels were added. The finer lymphatic fibres were given their knotty appearance by dripping white warm wax along a thin silk thread. the finer details were applied in paint. The bones were made of wax containing 'gilder's chalk' ground very finely and with colour added. When a transparent membrane was required, a marble table was kept at the right temperature with warm water; the wax was then poured and made extremely thin by means of a roll; several layers were thus applied, until the required transparency was obtained. When the model with all its final touches was completed, it was eventually covered with a film of copal for protection.

The workers were all specialists, in the sense that an expert on the circulatory system laid the veins and arteries, others the nerves, the lymphatic vessels, the viscera.

In the more delicate pieces, for example the small full-bodied models measuring about 60 cm, the method was slightly different. After making the model in clay, the mould was made in plaster in the usual way; then the interior of the mould was irrigated with a soft soap to block the pores, and was then smeared with a mixture of oil and lard. At this point, while still keeping the plaster mould opened in two halves, an extremely thin layer of wax, coloured like the surface, was spread inside, by means of a brush with long soft hairs; the wax had to be lukewarm (temperature tested on the cheek) and one continued in this way, with lukewarm wax, until the required thickness, 1 mm or less, had been obtained. To this first layer was added a second stronger layer, composed of a mixture of bee's wax and vegetable wax (Colophonian resin) at a slightly lower temperature and of a different

30

colour. According to the desired transparency, these thin layers were sometimes built up from as many as five or six separate applications of wax. At this point the mould was closed, leaving an outlet; then a third denser layer was trickled inside. When the whole had been well cooled, the mould was opened and the imperfections were removed with a lukewarm iron tool.

In conclusion, it is recorded that other small collections can be found elsewhere, in the Institutes of Human Anatomy of Padova, Cagliari and Bologna, of Pathological Anatomy at Florence and others. Some were ordered by Napoleon (1796) and sent to Paris but, because of some jealousy perhaps, they remained unpacked and were eventually sent to the School of Anatomy of Montpellier (1802). The Emperor of Austria Joseph II commissioned a great number of wax models for the Surgical Military Academy in Vienna. The order was too exacting for the Museum workshop and the Grand Duke refused it; Felice Fontana then took the appointment upon himself and gathered the necessary workers in his own house. The amazing work, over 1200 pieces, was completed in 5 years and in 1786 the great collection set off for Vienna through Italy and the Alps on mule back!

REFERENCES
Azzaroli M L 1975 *La Specola, The Zoological Museum of Florence University* (Firenze: Olschki) (Book prepared on the occasion of the 1st International Congress on Wax Modelling in Science and Art, Florence, June 1975.)
Berzi A, Cipriani C and Poggesi M 1980 'Florentine scientific museums' *J. Soc. Bibliogr. Natural History* **9** 413–25

Martin Luther on Medicine, Mathematics and Theology

Medicine makes people ill, mathematics makes them sad and theology makes them sinful.

A Plea for the Pigtail

The Chinese pigtail is an appendage which the progress of European civilisations now threatens with extinction. He maintains that the pigtail, like many other national customs, owed its origin to hygienic motives, and in one aspect formed the basis of China's ancient civilisation. He assures us that the effect of the pigtail is a more active circulation of the blood, which benefits the brain. He writes: 'The observations we hear now and then that Chinese without pigtails show less intelligence strikes me as not altogether unreasonable, as an active circulation of the blood will not fail to influence the nourishment and development of the brain.' He relates how the Chinese give special care to the head even of a newly born baby, and how it is shaved, and no cloth, cap, or soft pillow is allowed to interfere with the circulation of the scalp. When the child grows bigger, the hair is tied together in bunches, so as to expose the skin to the air, and thus promote perspiration. Later the hair is grown so as to form a pigtail, and superfluous hair is shaved away. The effect of the pigtail is a high and smooth forehead, and a face free from wrinkles; and so even old Chinese show smooth faces and a juvenile appearance. When rolled up on the top of the head, the pigtail acts as a substitute for a cap, and protects the head from the glare of the summer sun and the cold of winter. It also serves as a neckcloth and a pillow. As a cord, it is ever at hand to check haemorrhage. In addition to these virtues, the author attributes to it an inner and a moral meaning, for it is the symbol of the common nationality of 400 millions of people. Thus have Europeans, in dread of the power of China, adopted a method of protection by enticing the Chinese to become Europeans, and cut their pigtails off. This is the opinion of a European who, as we see, is more Chinese than John Chinaman himself. He neglects to remind us that the pigtail was only introduced by the Manchus somewhere about the middle of the seventeenth century of the Christian era, although it seems to be the fact that at an earlier date Chinese men let their hair grow long, and gathered it into a knot at the top. Still it remains for Dr Budberg to convince us that the European Delilah is really devising the ruin of the Chinese Samson by tonsorial methods.

REFERENCE
British Medical Journal 1912 **2** 1633–4

Spanish Proverb

El Médico lleva la plata, pero Dios es que sana. (The physician takes the fee, but God sends the cure.)

The Two-Headed Nightingale

(Courtesy Wellcome Institute Library, London.)

Fire Damage

World Medicine of 21 September 1977 reported that the following information had been given in the *Daily Telegraph*.

> A Dutch vet was fined £140 for burning down a farm with a jet of flame from the rear end of a cow. He lit a match to test the gas and the flame set alight to bales of hay, causing damage estimated at £45,000. The cow escaped with shock.

Barnum's Prize Ladies

(Courtesy Wellcome Institute Library, London.)

Anecdote on Dr Cunningham

Contributed by Alan Frank after an interview on BBC Radio London about *Mould's Medical Anecdotes*. It relates to a story told to keep students awake during lectures in Cambridge.

A woman patient told the eminent physician Dr Cunningham, author of the much-used manuals of dissection, that she had been given a digitalis examination by another doctor. 'I assume that he wore foxgloves, was Dr Cunningham's retort.

34

The Biddenden Maids

(Courtesy Wellcome Institute Library, London.)

35

(Courtesy Wellcome Institute Library, London.)

Hippocratic Hoax

There was published in 1958[1] in the student's club journal of the Welsh National School of Medicine, what purported to be a short Hippocratic text which had previously been overlooked by scholars and was stated to have been at one stage in the Library of the Church of Santa Eufrasia in Pisa. The journal editor described the author as a *special correspondent in New York* and the paper had all the outward signs of respectability with references, footnotes and, of course, the editor's backing. The text of this rare find dealt with many fields, including prognostics, epidemics, aphorisms, in the surgery, fractures and articulations and ancient medicine. The following are some of the words of wisdom from the pen of Hippocrates.

(*a*) Absence of respiration is a bad sign.

(*b*) It is unfavourable for the patient to be purple, especially if he is also cold. The physician should not promise a cure in such cases.

(*c*) Haemorrhoids are not improved by horseback riding or by riding on an ass.

(*d*) On the island of Tenebros, in the spring of the year, several maidens were attacked by swelling of the abdomen and absence of menstrual discharge. Giddiness, face flushed, absence of the membrane. A voyage to Asia was recommended. Complete crisis at the end of the ninth month.

(*e*) Life is short and the art is long; patients are inscrutable; their ignorance is impenetrable and their relatives impossible.

(*f*) Dislocation of the neck, which has been produced by a rope, cannot be treated with barley water.

(*g*) Where symptoms are severe and protracted, it is good if the patient's relatives are few, and best if they be absent altogether.

REFERENCE
[1] Gano S N 1958 'A gloss attributed to the Hippocratic School' *Leech* **4** 17–19

Anecdote of George James Guthrie, FRS Army Surgeon to Wellington

Guthrie (1795–1856) was a famous surgeon of the nineteenth century who was President of the Royal College of Surgeons three times

(1833, 1842, 1854) and surgeon to the Westminster Hospital 1827–43. In addition he had a very eventful medical career from the age of 13 until the year 1814 when the last battle of the Peninsula War was fought.

George James Guthrie, FRS.

At the age of 13 he was invited by Mr Rush, the Inspector General of the Army Hospitals, to become a 'surgeon's mate', and in 1800 went to the Army Hospital, York Hospital in Euston Square. But in 1801, Mr Keate the Surgeon-General refused to employ unqualified hospital mates any longer. Thus, Guthrie and his three other 'mates' were faced with a dilemma. The other three resigned, but Guthrie, at two days' notice, took the MRCS examination and passed. He was 16 years old. The Royal College of Surgeons shortly afterwards passed a regulation to prevent candidates acquiring the diploma before the age of 21. Guthrie was appointed Regimental Assistant Surgeon to 29th Foot and after service in North America went to the Peninsula with Wellington in 1808 and was present at the battles of Rolica and Vimeiro (where he was wounded in both legs by a musket ball).

On recovery he was at Talavera, Albuera (where there were 3000 wounded) and the sieges of Cuidad Rodrigo and Badajoz. After the battle of Salamanca his masterly handling of the wounded won him the approval of Wellington, who later appointed him Deputy-Inspector of Hospitals. He was also present in 1814 at the last battle of the Peninsula War, Toulouse, where he made a collection of specimens of gunshot wounds to bone: no doubt from the victims of Sir Thomas Picton's rash attack, whose bodies lying in their red tunics in the green water meadows led them to be called the 'Flowers of Toulouse'. The casualties that day were 3200 French and 4500 Allied soldiers, and it was after this battle that Napoleon abdicated and went into exile in Elba. Napoleon had in fact tried to commit suicide after the battle was lost, but the poison, prepared two years earlier for an emergency in Russia, was stale.

Guthrie was not rewarded very well, and, because of his youth, the medical authorities refused to gazette his appointment as Deputy-Inspector and he was placed on half pay. To improve his financial situation he managed to acquire two private patients in 1815. However, he was recalled to the colours for Waterloo (arriving the day after the battle) and it is recorded that neither of his two private patients ever spoke to him again!

REFERENCES
Humble J G and Hansell P 1974 *Westminster Hospital, 1716–1974* (London: Pitman Medical)
Longford E 1971 *Wellington, The Years of the Sword* (London: Panther Books)

Pliny on Doctors

Pliny the Elder (AD 23–79) commented on doctors when compiling his *Natural History*: 'There is no doubt that all these, in their hunt for popularity by means of some new gimmick, trafficked for it with our lives. This is the cause of those wretched, quarrelsome consultations at the bedside of the patients, when no doctor agrees with another, in case he may appear to acknowledge a superior. This is also the cause of that unfortunate epitaph on a tomb: 'He died from an overdose of doctors'. Medicine changes every day, again and again it is revamped, and we are swept along on the puffings of the best brains of Greece. It is obvious that anyone among them, who acquires the power of speaking, immediately assumes supreme control over our life and death, just as if thousands of people do not in fact live without doctors, though not without medicine, as the Roman people have done for more than six hundred years. The Roman people themselves were not slow in welcoming science—indeed, they were even greedy for medicine—until they tried it, and condemned it.'

Why Choose Anaesthetics or Dermatology?

'Anaesthetics' because: you can sit down during all operations and you never meet a patient who is awake.

'Dermatology' because:
(1) your patients never call you out at night;
(2) they never die;
(3) they keep on paying.

Excuses, Excuses!

Some of the replies from patients in response to a circular asking if they required transport to and from the chiropody clinic. (Contributed by Mr J M McGarry, FRCOG, Barnstaple.)

I am under the doctor and cannot breathe.
I can't walk to the bus stop and my wife is bent.
I can't use my legs or my wife's.
I cannot wait for a bus as it might rain.
I can't breathe and haven't done so for many years.
I am blind in one eye and my leg.
I live five miles from the clinic and postman says I should have it.
I have got arthritis and heart failure in both feet and knees.
I am unable to walk as my dog has died.
I have arthritis of the spine and can hardly walk into doors.
I suffer with my chest and have a job getting breath at the local shops.
I cannot walk up a hill unless it is down and the hill to the clinic is up.
I suffer from thyroid and cannot climb as I don't have a car.
I have not got a bus or a husband and my home help comes.
I cannot walk far because my husband is bedridden.
I haven't had my feet done for months but they are no better when I have been.
My husband is dead and will not bring me.
My wife must have transport as she is over 80 and drives me mad.

40

I must have your transport. We have a car but my husband is 76 and I
    haven't had it for a long time.
I can't walk any distance because I have a hip.
I must have transport as I have funny feet.
I cannot drive a car because I haven't got one.
My mother is 96 and must have a car as she has got long fingernails.
I want transport as bus drivers do funny things to me and make me
    feel queer, I am nearly 86.
If mother goes out alone she gets into trouble.
I hope you will still send your driver as my husband is quite useless.
I must have your man as I cannot go out or even do up my
    suspenders.
When your man brings me back will you ask him to drop me off at the
    White Swan.
I don't have a bus 83 years old.
I can come any time to suit you but not mornings as I don't feel too
    good. I can't come Monday or Wednesday as home help comes, and
    not Friday as the baker calls for his money. I can't come on Tuesday
    as my sister visits.

Surgeon's Hazards, Babylon, 1000 BC

As early as 1000 BC it has been recorded that successful operations for
cataract took place in Babylon. The fees were fixed by law and the
surgeon would receive 10 silver shekels for a patient who was a rich
freeman but only 2 silver shekels for a slave. These fees, however,
were for successful operations. Mistakes were more costly. If the
freeman lost the sight of his eye, then one of the surgeon's hands
would be cut off, whereas if it was the slave who was blinded, the
doctor had to provide a new slave for the owner.

Anecdote of Dr Gilmore and Dr Graham

Dr James Gilmore was the first patient to have one whole lung
removed surgically at a single operation.[1] This treatment was for
squamous cell carcinoma of the lung when he was 48 years old in 1933.
The surgeon was Dr Evarts Graham who, when he was positive that
the tumour was malignant, told Gilmore and described to him the
planned operation. Gilmore asked for a few days to go home and

arrange his affairs and included in this was the purchase of a cemetary lot. Most unusually, the patient also paid a visit to his dentist to fill some cavities that had been bothering him! Graham later said[2] in 1957 that Gilmore had told him that the visit to the dentist was to give him great assurance! The pneumonectomy was successful and Dr Gilmore died in 1963 at the age of 78 years: cause of death was cardio-renal disease. He outlived his surgeon by six years since Dr Graham died in 1957 of inoperable cancer of the lung.[3]

REFERENCES
[1] Graham E A and Singer J J 1933 'Successful removal of an entire lung for carcinoma of the bronchus' *J. Am. Med. Assoc.* **101** 1371–74
[2] Graham E A 1957 'A brief account of the development of thoracic surgery and some of its consequences' *Surg. Gynaecol. Obstet.* **104** 241–50
[3] Eloesser L 1970 'Milestones in chest surgery' *J. Thorac. Cardiovasc. Surg.* **60** 157–65

God and the Doctor

Contributed by Michael Aspel, 31 May 1984 on Capital Radio during an interview about *Mould's Medical Anecdotes*. Verse by John Owen (1560–1622)

> God and the doctor we alike adore
> But only when in danger and not before
> The danger o'er, both are requited
> God is forgotten and the doctor slighted

Australian Medicine Man with Magic Healing Crystal

This is a type of medical magic, seriously applied, which many primitive races practise after the ordinary domestic remedies have been used without much success. The healing crystal, the Oruncha, is invisible and imaginary, but this does not detract from its magic powers. The body markings are magical and represent healing crystals.

REFERENCE
Stubbs S G B and Bligh E W 1931 *Sixty Centuries of Health and Physik*
(London: Sampson Low, Marston & Co.)

Physician's Fees in St Louis, 1829

At a meeting of the medical faculty of the city of St Louis, held at the
City Hall on the 23rd day of November, 1829, the following
regulations for fees were unanimously entered into:

For the first visit in the city $1.00
For two or more visits to regular patients, per day $2.00
For a whole day's medical attention $10.00
For a night visit (expressly) after 9 o'clock $2.00
For a whole night's medical attention $10.00

43

For visit in the country, per mile $1.00
For consultation $5.00
For writing a prescription $1.00
For verbal prescription or advice $1.00
For treating syphilis $20.00
For treating gonorrhea $10.00
For natural labors, from .... $8.00 to $20.00
For preternatural, difficult, etc, labors .... $30.00 to $40.00
For amputating fingers, toes and other small members $10.00
For amputating arm, leg or thigh $50.00
For introducing catheter $5.00
For extracting tooth $1.00
For bleeding $1.00
For opening abscess .... From $1.00 to $2.00
For the operation for strangulated hernia $60.00
For operating for lithotomy .... From $100.00 to $200.00

REFERENCE
'One hundred years of medicine and surgery in Missouri' *St. Louis Star* 1900 pp 52–3

Confucius on Medicine

When Chi-sun Fei sent him medicine, he received it with a deep bow but said, 'since I do not recognise it, I will not put it in my mouth'.

One of the 450 sayings of Confucius (551–479 BC)

An Opinion on Quacks, 1714

Those who have little or no faith in the abilities of a quack will apply themselves to him, either because he is willing to sell health at a reasonable profit, or because the patient, like a drowning man, catches at every twig and hopes for relief from the most ignorant when the most able physicians give him none.

REFERENCE
The Spectator 26 July 1714

CIGARS DE JOY

GIVE IMMEDIATE

RELIEF IN CASES

OF ASTHMA, COUGH, BRONCHITIS, HAY-FEVER AND SHORTNESS OF BREATH.

One of these Cigarettes gives IMMEDIATE RE-LIEF in the worst attack of ASTHMA, HAY FEVER-CHRONIC BRONCHITIS, INFLUENZA, COUGH, and SHORTNESS OF BREATH, and their daily use effects a COMPLETE CURE. The contraction of the air tubes, which causes tightness of chest and difficulty of breathing, is at once lessened by inhaling the medi-cated smoke of the Cigarette, a free expectoration en-sues, and the breathing organs resume their natural action. Persons who suffer at night with COUGHING, PHLEGM, and SHORT BREATH, find them invalu-able, as they instantly check the spasm, promote sleep, and allow the patient to pass a good night.

These Cigarettes, invented by Mons. Joy, have been successfully tested and recommended by the Medical Profession for many years. They are perfectly harmless, and can be smoked by ladies, children, and the most delicate patients, as they are pleasant to use, and con-tain no substance capable of deranging the system.

Price **2s. 6d.** per box of 35, and may be obtained of all Chemists, or, post free, from WILCOX & CO., 336, OXFORD STREET, LONDON, on receipt of Stamps or P.O.O. NONE GENUINE UNLESS SIGNED ON BOX, E. W WILCOX.

(Courtesy Mary Evans Picture Library.)

Take a Wine-Moistened Topaz

The writings of ancient alchemists and philosophers such as Para-celsus, Van Helmont, Cornelius Agrippa and other students of the Caballa and Gnostics indicate the importance of gems in diagnosis and therapy. They considered that there was nothing purer than a precious stone because it was the product of a gradual process of purification and crystallisation going on in the mineral kingdom through long stages of evolution.

The medicinal powers of diamond—for good and bad—were widely accepted. In 1532, his doctors prescribed costly doses of powdered precious stones to cure a lingering ailment of the pontiff,

Clement VII. Much of the mixture was diamond. Unfortunately, it is on record that the patient died after the fourteenth spoonful. The Spanish favoured diamond dust for treatment of bladder trouble and the plague, with entirely predictable results.

A well known medieval gemmologist, Marbodus Redonensis, twelfth century Bishop of Rennes, commended the healing powers of topaz and the virtues of a green jasper amulet against fever and dropsy. He suggested amethyst for warding off drunkenness and emerald as a cure for epilepsy and malaria. Later, Paracelsus used powdered jacinth mixed with an equal amount of laudanum as a remedy for fevers of various origins.

Ruby has been claimed to be the most precious of the twelve stones created by God and this 'Lord of Gems' was placed on Aaron's neck by His command. It has always been held in high esteem by the Hindu people who consider that the glowing hue of the gem is an inextinguishable fire. Ruby was said to preserve the mental and bodily health of the wearer; it removed evil thoughts, and, although considered to be associated with passion, it was also thought to control amorous desires and to dispel pestilential vapours and reconcile disputes. Rubies were considered to be a remedy for haemorrhage and inflammatory disease. They were believed to confer invulnerability from wounds, but the Burmese said that it was not sufficient to wear the stones, but that they must be inserted into the flesh, becoming part of the wearer's body.

IN MEDICAL USE TODAY

Even in this day of men landing on the Moon, there is a hospital in India's state of Hyderabad which practises a Moslem system of medicine calling for the use of powdered gems. Entitled *Unani*, this system prescribes mixtures of oxidised jewels, dried fruit, honey, sugar and a variety of Indian spices. *Unani* practitioners claim that jewels provide chemicals in their purest form and have virtues beyond their chemical composition. Emeralds are recommended for ailments of the liver and kidneys, rubies for the heart, coral for asthma and the brain, diamonds for external use. Yet this is a modern, up-to-date hospital.

Among the *materia medica* of St Hildegard who lived in the tenth century was topaz to brighten dim vision. She advised her patients to rub their eyes with a wine-moistened topaz before retiring for the night. She also claimed that the same stone neutralised any liquid poison. The holy lady claimed that precious stones worked their medical wonders when merely held in the hand, grasped while making the Sign of the Cross, placed next to the skin, and breathed upon, held in the mouth (especially while fasting), or taken to bed to be warmed by the heat of the body. It was also the saint who suggested that epileptics cook their food only in water in which an agate had been soaking for three days.

Ancient physicians used gems both in diagnosis and healing paying particular regard to the 'dispositions' and 'moods' of the patient when tested against a gem.

RELATION OF GEMS TO DISPOSITIONS AND MOODS

Amethyst. Regarded as the emblem of self-control and self-discipline. It was said to preserve the wearer from intoxication, both alcoholic and psychic, thus keeping the mind and body clear and well balanced.

Agate. Worn as a charm against scorpions and spiders. People who found the radiations of the stone disturbing were usually found to be prone to fits of anger, bad temper and jealousy.

Turquoise. Associated with health and the preservation and restoration of vital energy. It was also given as a symbol of conjugal fidelity and chastity. If this stone was worn by a person suffering from a chronic condition, malignant disease or infection of the blood, it was reputed to lose its lustre, the blue or blue-green colour changing to a muddy, dull brownish moss-green.

Lapus-lazuli. Used medicinally in a finely pulverised form, mixed with honey, as a remedy for sterility. The ancients considered that people who are emotionally unbalanced and very sensual will not be able to keep this stone long—always losing it.

Opal. Medieval philosophers praised this gem very highly, considering it conducive to idealism and impersonality, taking the wearer into abstract lands away from the material sphere of life.

Coral. Although not a true gem Paracelsus recommended red coral as a remedy against melancholy and evil influences. Brown coral, according to him, should not be worn as it attracts undesirable forces.

Amber. Fossilised resin of coniferous vegetation of the Tertiary period. With its high electrical properties, it was worn against the body to prevent the wearer from losing nervous energy.

PREPARATION

For healing purposes, gems were used in the following ways:
(*a*) The gem was soaked in pure water, kept in a glass or crystal

container and exposed to sunlight from the east. The irradiated water was then given as a drink or preserved with the admixture of a little wine and given in drops.

(*b*) Some of the gems were pulverised into a fine powder which was then mixed with honey and given internally, or mixed with tallow (mutton fat) and used as an ointment. Or it was mixed with a little water into a thin paste which was painted over the affected part. Pulverised jet mixed with honey was given as a remedy for flatulence.

DIAGNOSIS

For diagnosis, certain gems were related to various parts of the body:

Amber	Nervous system
Amethyst	Lymph and glands
Agate	Stomach and inflammations
Alabaster	Skin
Beryl	Eyes
Carbuncle	Blood stream
Cornelian	Chest and heart
Coral	Abdomen
Garnet	Liver and gall bladder
Jade	Kidneys
Jet	Intestines
Lapus lazuli	Reproductive organs
Malachite	Eye lids
Moonstone	Throat
Opal	Spleen
Rose quartz	Head—Brain—Epilepsy
Topaz	Rectum and bladder
Turquoise	Blood purifier and a tonic
Tourmaline	Spinal column

The sixteenth century physician and pharmacist, Bulleyn, a cousin of Henry VIII's wife, Anne Boleyn, wrote a prescription containing 'two drachms of white perles; two little peeces of saphyre; jacinthe, corneline, emeraulds, granettes, of each an ounce; redded corrall, amber, shaving of ivory, of each two drachms; thin peeces of gold and sylver, of each half a scruple.' These very expensive prescriptions were in common use against disease and poison.

In today's world of wonder drugs and medical miracles, one wonders what the Ministry would reply to a doctor who recommended ruby for a National Health patient and how the charges would be met.

REFERENCE
Glogger T J 1971 *History of Medicine* **3** 29–30

Toothache in the Third Century AD?

The illustration is of a funerary slab, probably of the third century AD in ancient Rome. It shows a doctor examining the face of a woman patient. The scene below may represent mourners at her deathbed.

(Courtesy Mansell Collection.)

Oscar Wilde's Dying Words

I expect I shall have to die beyond my means (said after accepting a glass of champagne).

49

Napoleon on Doctors

Doctors will have more lives to answer for in the next world than even we generals.

Medical Ants

The closing of surgical wounds using catgut or thread sutures is widely known but a forerunner of these materials will come as a surprise to most people. In an early medical text by Albucasis[1] it is stated in Latin: 'Deinde aggrega duo labia vulneris et pone fornicam unam ex eis que habebant os apertum super duo labia vulneris'. This refers to sewing up the colon with a kind of ant with a big head. As soon as the ant has closed up its mouth, the head is cut off and it rests attached to the wound. Immediately a second ant is used for the following suture, and so on, until the entire wound is closed. The method had previously been described by the ancient Hindu surgeon Susruta who recommended the heads of red ants, and this practice was even followed in the nineteenth century[2] in the war between the Greeks and the Turks in 1821 when Turkish surgeons followed this method.

REFERENCES
[1] De Lint J G 1927 'The treatment of the wounds of the abdomen in ancient times' *Annals of Medical History* **7** 403–7
[2] Gurlt E J 1898 *Geschichteder Chirurgie, Berlin* **1** 97

Pour the Medicine Over the Patient's Head!

In addition to poultices and drugs to cure irritated membranes, to reduce swellings, to open the bowels and to get rid of wind, the ancient Babylonians and Assyrians also recommended such curious remedies as pouring concoctions over a patient's head. An example is for a man with cramps: *either*

Let that man sit down, with his feet under him, pour boiled . . . and cassia juice over his head and he will recover.

or

Let him kneel and pour cold water on his head.

The choice was usually between a warm and a cold douche and if one afforded no relief then the other could be tried. A variation of the treatment for cramps included a massage to stimulate the circulation, but it sounded worse for the patient than the original cramps!

Place his head downwards and his feet under him, manipulate his back with the thumb, saying 'be good', manipulate his arms 14 times and his head 14 times, rolling him on the ground.

The address 'be good' was apparently directed at the demon causing the cramps. Why 14 was a magic number is not known.

REFERENCE
Jastrow M 1917 'Babylonian-Assyrian Medicine' *Annals of Medical History* **1** 241

Remarkable Prevention of Poaching

A gentleman of Hampshire, who was in the habit of being robbed almost every night by poachers, adopted a novel and effectual mode of putting an end to this depredation. He went to London, purchased a man's leg at a hospital, and on his return had it hung up near the next place of public meeting, with a label attached to it, stating it had been caught on his grounds, and requesting the right owner would send for it. This had such an effect that he has not since been robbed.

REFERENCE
John Bull Newspaper No 10 18 February 1821 p 80

Gravestone Inscription in America's Rural South

I told you I was sick.

'Sorry Sir, But What Your Wife Wants is Not Available on Prescription'

One of a series of drawings by Mr Harald Nymark for the posters of H Lundbeck A/S Copenhagen.

An Experiment with Rats

The investigator reported that one third of the rats were improved on the experimental medication, one third remained the same, and the other one third could not be reported on because that rat got away.

Edwin Bidwell Wilson (1879–1964)

'In My Spare Time I Shoe Horses'

Another Nymark drawing for a Lundbeck poster.

Saint Who's?

By my last reckoning there were 160 hospitals in Britain named after a saint. St Mary has easily the largest number (26) with St John (13) in second place and St George and St Luke jointly third, with nine each. Others are St Andrew and St Michael (six each); Anne, Margaret, James, and Peter (five each); Paul and David (four each); Nicholas, Thomas, Clement, Lawrence, Leonard, and Catherine (three each); Matthew, Stephen, Bartholomew, Francis, Joseph and Martin (two each). Thirty two saints patronise just one hospital—Aldhelm, Anthony, Audrey, Augustine, Barnabus, Blazey, Cadoc, Chad, Charles, Christopher, Crispin, Ebba, Editha, Edmund, Edward, Faith, Giles, Helen, Helier, Hilda, Mark, Monica, Olave, Oswald, Pancras, Philip, Saviour, Theresa, Vincent, Wilfrid, Woolas and Wulstan.

These simple facts give us considerable opportunity for speculation. When there are several saints with the same name which is the one concerned? Why was he or she chosen? Does the saint have any special medical connection? And who were some of the saints on the list with unfamiliar names?

It seems a reasonable assumption that most if not all the St Marys refer to the Blessed Virgin, pre-eminent among the saints although with no medical association; St Mary Magdalene is a possibility for one or two but she has no medical association either.

There are three main contenders for the hospitals named St John. Either the Baptist or the Evangelist may be intended but St John of God is the strongest candidate although he is usually given his complete title to distinguish him from the other two. He was a fifteenth century Portugese who fought for years in the Spanish army before becoming fired with religious zeal. Unable to reach North Africa, where he hoped to die a martyr's death ransoming slaves, he became a highly successful seller of religious books and pictures. Then he went mad, gave away his books, and ran wildly through the streets. Eventually he recovered and devoted the rest of his life to helping the sick.

PATRONESS OF CHILDBIRTH

Several St Margarets contest the five hospitals with this name but the favourite is St Margaret of Antioch. She was a mythical figure whose legend tells of her refusal to marry the pagan governor of Antioch since she was an avowed Christian virgin. She was tortured in a variety of ways and at one point was swallowed by a dragon which found her indigestible and burst asunder. She became the patroness of childbirth because of a promise made before she died that women who invoked her would be safe during pregnancy and labour. The Holy See supressed her cult in 1969 but her name lives on. One St Margaret's Hospital, however, in Auchterarder, Scotland, surely suggests a dedication to St Margaret of Scotland, grand daughter of Edmund Ironside and Queen to King Malcolm III. She was a woman of saintly behaviour and disposition who bore her husband eight children. One of them, King David of Scotland, also became a saint, but it seems unlikely that any of the four hospitals which bear that name refer to him. All are in Wales and are surely named after the patron saint of that country who flourished in south Wales in the sixth century.

We have only one small clue to suggest which St James—James the Greater or James the Less—deserves the title to four hospitals. James the Greater used to be invoked for the cure of rheumatism although there is nothing in his life or legend to suggest that he suffered from it.

Three hospitals are named St Thomas but after whom—St Thomas the Apostle, Thomas Aquinas, Thomas of Canterbury, or even Thomas of Hales or Thomas of Hereford? If we are to be guided by medical considerations the apostle and Thomas Becket are the favourites. St Thomas, the twin, who refused to believe in the risen Lord until he could put his finger in the marks of the nails and his hand in Christ's side, used to be invoked for the cure of blindness and eye disorders because of the spiritual blindness he showed on that occasion. In this sense, therefore, we might regard him as a specialist but St Thomas of Canterbury was clearly a general practitioner since a prodigious number of cures from a wide variety of disorders were attributed to drinking the water of St Thomas—a large volume of water into which had been sprinkled tiny particles of the dried blood of the saint.

St Catherine of Alexandria is more likely to be intended as patron of three hospitals bearing her name than St Catherine of Genoa or of Siena. Like Margaret of Antioch, Catherine of Alexandria was a mythical figure whose cult was also suppressed by the Holy See in 1969. Her legend tells us that she, like Margaret, refused to marry a high-ranking pagan suitor since she had dedicated her life to Almighty God. Fifty philosophers were called in to show her the error of her Christian ways but she confounded them and many who heard the debate became Christian. She was condemned to die on a huge spiked wheel (the Catherine wheel of 5 November) but the wheel collapsed killing her torturers, and thousands more became Christians. Finally, she was beheaded when milk—the milk of human kindness—spouted from her body instead of blood, leading to her patronage of nurses.

The search for a specific medical connection in the many other hospital patrons reveals surprisingly few—Anthony, Chad, Christopher, Edmund, George, Giles, Leonard, Luke and Oswald.

ST ANTHONY OF EGYPT OR OF PADUA?

Two St Anthonys, each with a medical association, contest one hospital at Cheam. St Anthony of Egypt was the archetypal desert hermit who gave away all his money and lived in solitude, enduring formidable privations and temptations until his death at the age of 99.

Ergot poisoning was once called St Anthony's fire, an association which came about because, in the Middle Ages, the monks of the Order of Hospitallers of St Anthony opened hospitals with red painted walls for sufferers from the disease, in which affected fingers and toes burn like fire. The original name was holy fire (*ignis sacer*) before St Anthony had his name attached. Representations of the saint show him with a bell, denoting his hermit status, and a pig since the monks of the order were allowed to let their pigs roam the streets. St Anthony of Padua, famous as a finder of lost articles, used to be invoked also for the cure of infertility, an association hard to understand. But which is patron of Cheam Hospital?

An equally puzzling link with infertility is found in St Edmund who was also invoked by barren women. He was King of the East Angles and was martyred by the Danes in 869. On 20 November, his feast day, it was at one time the custom for infertile women to walk alongside a white bull stroking its flanks until they reached the monastery gates when the women went inside to the saint's shrine to offer prayers that they might conceive. But this does not explain why St Edmund's Hospital is in Northampton.

More geographically appropriate is a hospital named after St Chad, the first Bishop of Lichfield, in Birmingham. It is also medically appropriate since, in former times, pilgrims visiting his shrine could put their hands through a little aperture in the wall, take some dust from within, sprinkle it into water, and give it to an invalid to drink with every expectation of cure.

We have seen a similar condition already with the water of St Thomas and we meet it again with St Oswald who has a hospital at Ashbourne. Oswald, King of Northumbria, was killed fighting the heathen King of Mercia, Penda, in 642. The Venerable Bede describes several miracles of healing near his grave and the cure of a man from the plague after he had drunk water into which had been placed a fragment of the stake which had impaled the severed head of the saint.

Plague also has an association with St Christopher, the patron of travellers who has a hospital at Fareham. He used to be invoked for protection against plague, tempest and flood, all hazards which a traveller in former times could expect to encounter.

It is not surprising that all nine hospitals named after St George are in England. Apart from being the national patron he is also patron of soldiers which explains why he was invoked for the cure of skin disease. Serious cutaneous sores and skin eruptions severely troubled soldiers in former times so the association is not surprising. All we know of St George is that he was a soldier killed in Palestine in the second century. The story of his encounter with the dragon is entirely mythical.

LEPERS, NURSING MOTHERS AND CRIPPLES

St Giles has, nowadays, only one hospital dedicated to him and that is in London. At one time, however, when lepers were common, leper hospitals were named after him. He is patron saint of the unlikely combination of lepers, nursing mothers and cripples, perhaps one reason why his church in London is at Cripplegate. His legend tells, how, while living in the forest in the south of France, he was fed for a time by the milk of a hind—hence the nursing mothers. One day a hunting party pursued the hind and an arrow intended for it wounded the saint instead—hence the cripples. But we are in the dark about the lepers.

St Leonard, like St Giles, was a forest hermit, in which unlikely setting he became one of the patron saints of childbirth. The story goes that he was visited by King Clovis whose wife, heavy with child, was with him. She was safely delivered, thanks to St Leonard, but whether he acted as midwife or interceded with God on her account we do not know. He got a most original grateful patient present none the less—as much land as he could ride round in one night on a donkey. the animal covered so much ground that the saint was able to build the Abbey of Noblac on it.

We know from St Paul's Epistle to the Colossians that St Luke was a physician—the only one among the group of hospital patrons. Strangely he is almost always shown in hagiographic art in another guise—painting a picture of the Blessed Virgin with his emblem, an ox, close by. He is of course one of the patron saints of doctors but artists claim his as their patron also.

We will find few medical connections among the other patrons. Some have a simple geographical connection with a local saint. Frome, for example, has St Aldhelm's Hospital named for an abbot of Malmesbury and bishop of Wessex who died in 709; St Blazey, an early Cornish saint, has a hospital at Par bearing his name; St Cadoc, a sixth century saint from south Wales has a hospital at Caerleon, and his father, St Woolas, one at Newport; St Wulstan, the eleventh century Bishop of Worcester, has a hospital at Malvern, St Augustine, one at Canterbury, and St Hilda, abbess of a nunnery at Hartlepool in the seventh century has a hospital there; St Edith, or Editha, of Polesworth has given her name to a hospital at nearby Tamworth and St Wilfred to one at Ripon where he was abbot in the seventh century.

There are some patronages, however, which defy any such geographical explanation. Why does St Helier, the first martyr of Jersey, have a hospital in London; St Ebba, who was abbess of the nunnery of Coldingham on the remote Northumbrian coast, one at Epsom; or St Edmund of the East Angles one at Northampton?

Northampton, however, has one of the most delightfully original dedications in St Crispin's Hospital. The town is famous for its shoes and St Crispin and his brother St Crispinian are the patron saints of shoemakers since, to avoid taking alms from those to whom they preached, they supported themselves by their trade as cobblers.

With this ingenious dedication in mind is it too much to hope that future National Health Service hospitals—if any are built—might be more suitably named? Surely we need a children's hospital named after St Elmo, invoked for the cure of colic in children in the mistaken belief that he was martyred by having his intestines wound on to a windlass; and ear, nose and throat hospital named for St Blaise, the patron saint of throats; a mental hospital for St Vitus, invoked for the cure of mental disorder, epilepsy and possession by devils; a cancer hospital called after St Peregrine, a thirteenth century monk miraculously cured from a repulsive cancer on his foot the night before he was to have it amputated; and eye hospital called after St Lucy, the principal patron of the blind; and a dental hospital for St Apollonia, invoked for the cure of toothache.

And if the acquired immune deficiency syndrome (AIDS) ever becomes the scourge many fear and a hospital is built for its sufferers may it please be called St Fiacre's Hospital? St Fiacre was a sixth century Irish missionary who went to Gaul where he set up a hospice for the poor and sick but would never let a woman enter it. He was invoked for the cure of venereal disease.

REFERENCE
Dewhurst, Sir John 1986 *Br. Med. J.* **293** (December) 1618–21

Caesarean Section by the Patient Herself

Cases of Caesarean section by the patient herself are most curious, but may be readily believed if there is any truth in the reports from savage tribes. In 1884 there was an account of a successful case performed, with preservation of the lives of both mother and child, by a native African in Kahura, Uganda. The young girl operated in the crudest manner, the haemorrhage being check by a hot iron. The sutures were made by means of seven thin, hot iron spikes, resembling acupressure-needles, closing the peritoneum and skin. The wound healed in eleven days and the mother made a complete recovery.

An earlier case, described in the *London Medical Journal* of 1785, was of a negro woman who, being unable to bear the pains of labour any longer, took a sharp knife and made a deep incision in her belly—deep enough to wound the buttocks of her child, and extracted the child, placenta and all. A negro horse-doctor was called, who sewed the wound up in a manner similar to the way dead bodies are closed.

REFERENCE
Gould G M and Pyle W L 1900 *Anomalies and Curiosities of Medicine* (Philadelphia: Saunders)

John Shaw Billings on Statistics

Statistics are somewhat like old medical journals, or like revolvers in newly opened mining districts. Most men rarely use them, and find it troublesome to preserve them so as to have them easy of access; but when they do want them, they want them badly.

REFERENCE
Medical Record 1889 **36** 589

Somerset Maugham on Training

I do not know a better training for a writer than to spend some years in the medical profession.

Childbirth in Sicily

Nineteenth-century votive pictures. Thanksgiving after a successful operation and safe delivery in childbirth, Ethnographic Museum, Palermo, Sicily. (Courtesy Wellcome Institute Library, London.)

Pompeian Surgery and Surgical Instruments

POMPEII AND HERCULANEUM

The Romans occupied Campania in 88 BC, and thereafter Pompeii takes its place in Roman history, and is frequently mentioned by Seneca, Pliny and other contemporary writers. Toward the close of Nero's reign—that is to say, in the year AD 63—the whole region was visited by severe earthquakes, which made such a havoc that the cities were deserted for several years. The rebuilding of Pompeii appears to have been begun about AD 69, ten years before its final destruction, which took place on the 23 November AD 79 and appears to have commenced in the afternoon. Although Herculaneum and Pompeii were destroyed by the same eruption, they were destroyed in quite different ways. The former was filled up by a flow of warm muddy water, which filled it with a soft paste; and subsequent eruptions have covered it with molten lava no less than eleven times, rendering excavation exceedingly difficult and costly. Pompeii, on the other hand, was covered with loose ashes and pumice-stone, which were ejected from the volcano to a considerable height and blown into the city by the violent northwesterly gale which Pliny tells us was raging at that time. In short, Pompeii can be excavated with a trowel, but it takes a chisel to make an impression on Herculaneum.

The streets of the uncovered city of Pompeii bring vividly to the mind of the visitor the life, works, virtues, and vices of its former inhabitants. The old aqueduct that supplied the city with pure water from the mountains is well preserved and remains as one of the marvels of engineering of that time. The pavements of the streets can compare favorably with those of our day. The bare walls of public and private buildings testify to the unrivalled perfection masonry had attained at that day. The crude stone mills operated by human power furnished the city with flour, which in the adjacent bakery was converted into bread.

The enormous wine-jugs, so numerous in places where wine was sold and drunk, remain as lasting mementoes that the Pompeians were by no means prohibitionists. The numerous houses of prostitution, both public and private, remain as silent witnesses of a vice which appeared to have been unusually prevalent at that time. The capacious forum, amphitheatre, comic and tragic theatres that remain in a wonderful state of preservation, show that the people of that day—male and female, old and young—enjoyed the glittering stage and the bloody contests of the gladiators. The public bath-house is a marvel of its kind, and it is doubtful if in its artistic design and luxury it could be duplicated today. The private dwellings are all constructed on the same plan—masterpieces of comfort and sanitary construction. The numerous fountains furnished pure water for beast and man. The temple of Esculapius is one of the prominent landmarks of the former city, and fortunately time and the elements have dealt gently with its precious contents. In the centre of the capacious anteroom stands the altar of pure marble, beautifully carved, at which the priests of old worshipped in the interests of suffering humanity. It is here where the sick, the maimed and the injured sought relief.

A walk through the narrow, stone-paved streets of the uncovered part of the ruins of Pompeii is necessarily attended with serious thoughts of the past and present. The wider streets show deep grooves made by the chariot-wheels, while the narrower streets were reserved for pedestrians. The one-story buildings, both public and private, show a singular uniformity in their construction—evidence that the Pompeian architects and builders had in view more the comfort and health of their occupants than a desire to exhibit their talent. The many shops in the principal street were the homes and business places of merchants who supplied the citizens with the luxuries and necessities of life. A large building on the corner of two streets served as a drug-store, where crude drugs were dealt out to those in need of remedial agents. The proprietor of this primitive pharmacy—living, as he did, next door to a public house of prostitution—in order to protect himself and family against intrusion of an undesirable nature, found it necessary to place above the entrance a sign to indicate to the prospective customer the legitimate character of his business, and to direct him properly if he was in search of pleasure.

SURGICAL INSTRUMENTS

These instruments were found in a house which has since been called the 'Surgeon's House'. They are made of bronze, and some of them show a high degree of artistic workmanship. Some of them show the destructive effect of heat and oxidation, while others are in a state of excellent preservation, as will be seen from the illustrations. The illustrations are taken from specimens from the Naples Museum.

(*a*) Actual cautery. Length 10 in.

(*b*) Bivalve speculum working on a central pivot. Length 6 in. Width, when open, $2\frac{1}{2}$ in.

(*c*) Scissors with a spring-like shears. Length 4 in.

(*d*) A male catheter which is almost a facsimile of the one devised by J L Petit in the last century. At the closed end is an eye, as in the modern instrument. Length $10\frac{1}{2}$ in.

(*e*) Hook. Length 6 in.

(*f*) Point of injection-syringe, with eight small perforations near the distal end. The other end was, no doubt, filled with a syringe. Length 6 in.

(*g*) Pompeian forceps, formed of two branches, crossing and working on a pivot. Each branch is fitted with with an engine-turned handle and a spoon shaped blade. A powerful forceps, undoubtedly used for the extraction of foreign bodies. Length 8 in.

(*h*) Forceps with serrated bite. Length $4\frac{1}{2}$ in.

(*i*) Cupping-glass of bronze. Height 6 in, diameter 3 in.

(*j*) Medicine-box with medicines, 5×3 in.

(*k*) Spatula for mixing ointments. Length 7 in.

(*l*) Lancet for bleeding. Length 5 in.

(*m*) Fleam for bleeding horses. Length $5\frac{1}{2}$ in.

(*n*) Forceps. Length $4\frac{1}{2}$ in.

(*o*) Toothed dissecting-forceps with the engraved name, A. C. A. A: G. L. V. S. F. Length $7\frac{1}{2}$ in.

(*p*) Trocar for tapping, with a hole at the end for the escape of the fluid. Length 5 in.

63

(*q*) Small spoon with bone handle, ending in the head of a ram. Length 5½ in.

(*r*) Female catheter. Length 4 in.

(*s*) Bistoury, the blade oxidised and the handle in bronze. Length 5¾ in.

(*t*) Trivalve speculum, an instrument which, like the bivalve and the quadrivalve, has been much discussed by archaeologists and physicians. It is composed of three valves standing at right angles to the rest of the instrument, and jointly dependent on one another in the expansion transmitted only to one of them. By turning the screw one valve is drawn nearer the operator, and this forces the other two to open in a sidelong direction. The instrument can be held by the two curved handles with the left hand, while the right hand turn the screw. Length 8¼ in.; widest expansion of the two valves 1½ in.

(*u*) Spatula. Length 7 in.

(*v*) A metallic case containing surgical instruments. Length 8 × ¾ in.

These are some of the most important instruments found in the ruins of Pompeii, and which were employed by our ancestors two thousand years ago in the practice of surgery. I searched carefully, but without avail, for traces of needles or something else which would indicate that at that time wounds were sutured. The collection contains no saws, trephines, chisels or any other instruments for operations upon bones. All of the instruments with the exception of the specula and catheters are diminutive in size as compared with the same instruments of less remote and modern times. The absence of saws and chisels is noteworthy, as among the agricultural instruments these tools are represented by specimens of a high degree of perfection.

In the writings of Hippocrates raspatories, mallet and trephine are mentioned, and consequently must have been used in operations upon bones other than those of the skull. Hippocrates gives very minute directions as to the use of the trephine in the treatment of fractures of the skull:

> With regard to trepanning, when there is a necessity for it, the following particulars should be known: If you have had the management of the case from the first, you must not at once saw the bone down to the meninx, for it is not proper that the membrane should be laid bare and exposed to injuries for a length of time, as in the end it may become fungous. And there is another danger if you saw the bone down to the meninx and remove it at once, lest in the act of sawing you should wound the meninx. But in trepanning, when only a very little of the bone remains to be sawed through, and the bone can be moved, you must desist from sawing, and leave the bone to fall out of itself. For to a bone not sawed through, and where a portion is left of the

sawing, no mischief can happen; for the portion now left is sufficiently thin. In other respects you must conduct the treatment as may appear suitable to the wound, and in trepanning you must frequently remove the trepan, on account of the heat in the bone, and plunge it into cold water. For the trepan, being heated by running round, and heating and drying the bone, burns it and makes a larger piece of bone around the sawing to drop off than would otherwise do. And if you wish to saw at once down to the membrane and then remove the bone, you must also in like manner frequently take out the trepan and dip it into cold water. But if you have not charge of the treatment from the first, but undertake it from another after a time, you must saw the bone at once down to the meninx with a serrated trepan, and in doing so must frequently take out the trepan and examine with a sound, and otherwise along the track of the instrument. For the bone is much sooner sawn through, provided there be matter below it and in it, and it often happens that the bone is more superficial, especially if the wound is situated in that part of the head where the bone is rather thinner than in other places. But you must take care where you apply the trepan and see that you do so only where it appears to be particularly thick, and, having fixed the instrument there, that you frequently make examinations and endeavour by moving the bone to bring it up. Having removed it, you must appply the other suitable remedies to the wound. And if, when you have the management of the treatment from the first, you wish to saw through the bone at once and remove it from the membrane, you must in like manner examine the track of the instrument frequently with the sound, and see that it is fixed on the thickest part of the bone, and endeavour to remove the bone by moving it about. But if you use a perforator you must not penetrate to the membrane, if you operate on a case which you have had the charge of from the first, but must leave a thin scale of bone, as described in the process of sawing.

As Hippocrates at one time lived and practised in Athens during a great epidemic, it appears strange that his teachings in reference to the treatment of injuries of the skull should not have reached Pompeii, as evidenced by the absence of trepans and other bone-instruments in the 'House of the Surgeons'.

If we judge the worth of the Pompeian surgeon from the collection of instruments he left behind him, it is evident that bloody operations were confined to bleeding, cupping, extraction of foreign bodies and opening of abscesses. The metallic medicine-box, the spatula and spoon indicate that the surgeons of that time made free use of medicines and ointments in the treatment of injuries and disease. The instruments and implements of wood, splints, etc, were of course destroyed by fire and heat, and their absence in the collection leaves undoubtedly a large gap in the surgical resources of the Pompeian surgeon.

SURGEON'S HOUSE

The surgeon's house does not differ from the private houses in its vicinity. It is roofless like the rest, all that remains being the bare walls. It is here that most of the surgical instruments were found. This house was undoubtedly occupied by the principal surgeon of Pompeii, who ministered to those in need of surgical aid. It is here that bleeding and cupping were practised for all kinds of ills, real and imaginary. It is difficult to imagine what transpired from day to day. That the surgeon was a busy man there can be but little doubt. Competition was then not as active and pressing as it is now, and it is therefore safe to assume that the capacious waiting-room was crowded day after day by patients anxious to be bled, cupped or burned. These bare walls, if they could talk, could tell of many sad and exciting scenes. Fainting from loss of blood and writhing under the actual cautery, must have been frequent and familiar sights. How often the neighbourhood must have been disturbed by the cries of the suffering and the shrieks of the tortured! How often the atmosphere and adjacent streets must have been stifled with the smell of burned human flesh! Let us hope that the master escaped, leaving in his haste his instruments of skill and torture as lasting mementoes of his so suddenly interrupted professional career. The house is deserted and silent now, a permanent reminder of the great antiquity of the art of surgery. If the last representative of Pompeian surgery could return today and behold the improvements in surgery which have been made since his time, he would indeed be astonished and amazed. What would be his surprise if he could visit one of our modern hospitals and inspect an aseptic operating-room. He would find his old occupation gone. No need now for lancet, cupping-glass and actual cautery. He would find the science of surgery developed to a wonderful degree of perfection and its practice in consonance with its principles. He could make use of anaesthesia to prevent pain, Esmarch's bandage to guard against haemorrhage and operate under aseptic precautions to protect accidental and intentional wounds against complications the treatment of which made up a large part of the work of the ancient surgeon. He would perhaps be astonished to learn that since Pompeii was buried surgery not only came to a standstill, but retrograded for centuries, and that its present state of perfection is owing largely to the improvements and advancements made during the present century. Let us not forget, however, that our colleagues of the distant past, possessed of a primitive knowledge of anatomy, physiology and pathology, and armed with few and imperfect instruments to practise their art, laboured faithfully in the interest of suffering humanity, and unquestionably did much toward prolonging the lives and adding to the comfort and happiness of those who were entrusted to their care.

Bas relief from Pompeii of Nestor healing Machaon. (Courtesy Mansell Collection.)

POMPEIAN SURGERY

There can be but little doubt that the Pompeian surgeons practised surgery in accordance with the teaching of Hippocrates, who is justly entitled to be called the father of medicine, and was born on the island of Cos in 450 BC; hence his lifework was contemporaneous with the early history of Pompeii. It is not difficult to conceive that his teachings penetrated to this city, or that some of its surgeons might have been his pupils. In all probability, Pompeian surgery was Hippocratic surgery. As has been remarked before, the instruments which have been recovered from its ruins so far seem to indicate that no major operations were performed at that time, and that the surgeon's work was limited to cupping, bleeding, the treatment of injuries and the performance of minor operations. The discovery of a number of very ingenious specula in the 'House of the Surgeon' furnishes us with positive evidence that at that time gynaecology was not practised as a specialty, but constituted a legitimate part of the surgeon's work. Considering the character of the moral atmosphere of Pompeii, it is not astonishing to learn that diseases of the genito-urinary organs taxed the ingenuity and occupied much of the time and attention of its surgeons, as shown by the different kinds of specula then in use and the wonderfully perfect construction of the male and female catheter. The numerous wine-shops and houses of prostitution, private and public, that constitute such a conspicuous part of the ruins of Pompeii, stand as lasting monuments of the debauchery and licentiousness of its former inhabitants, and furnish a satisfactory explanation of the prevalence of genito-urinary diseases among males and females, and which so often necessitated the services of a surgeon. The fleam for bleeding horses found in the instrumentarium of the Pompeian surgeon goes to show that he extended his sphere of usefulness to the domestic animals, which furnished him with an additional field for observation and undoubtedly added materially to his income. That the surgeon of Pompeii was a man of means and good social position is amply testified to by the size and location of his house. This house is capacious, and is located in the aristocratic part of the city. A liberal income undoubtedly rewarded his labours and placed him in a position to enjoy the luxuries of life, which seems to have been the main object in life of the mass of the people at that time. The existence of a separate house occupied as a pharmacy shows that the people then, as now, had great faith in the healing powers of herbs and drugs, and the medicine-box found in the 'Surgeon's House' was replenished from time to time from this source, and its contents were undoubtedly frequently made use of by the surgeon in the practice of his profession.

REFERENCE
Adapted from Senn N 1895 'Pompeiian surgery and surgical instruments' *Medical News* **67** (28 December) 701–8

Cure for a Babylonian Hangover

The following is surely one of the most ancient remedies for the after-effects of a good night out on the bottle!

> If a man has drunk unmixed wine and has a severe headache, he forgets his words, his speech is heavy, his mind is clouded, his eyes are set, take (eleven plants are enumerated), mix them with oil and wine, let him drink before the approach of evening, and in the morning before anyone has kissed him.

REFERENCE
Jastrow M 1917 'Babylonian–Assyrian medicine' *Annals of Medical History* **1** 243

FREE TRIALS

AT 27, PRINCES STREET, HANOVER SQUARE, LONDON, W.

THE

CARBOLIC SMOKE BALL

WILL

POSITIVELY
CURE

COLDS

COLD IN THE HEAD

COLD ON THE CHEST

CATARRH

ASTHMA

BRONCHITIS

HOARSENESS

LOSS OF VOICE

INFLUENZA

HAY FEVER

THROAT DEAFNESS

SORE THROAT

SNORING

CROUP

WHOOPING COUGH

NEURALGIA

HEADACHE

For Inhalation only.

For Inhalation only.

This Infallible Remedy is Used by

Marchioness of Bath.
Marchioness of Conyngham.
Marchioness de Sain.
Countess of Dudley.
Countess Dowager of Meath.
Countess of Enniskillen.
Countess of Ravensworth.
Countess of Lanesborough.
Countess of Aberdeen.
Countess of Home.
Countess of Elgin.
Countess of Chichester.
Countess of Hardwicke.
Countess of Carnwath.
Countess Manvers.

Countess Ferrers.
Viscountess Cranbrook
Dowager Viscountess Downe.
Baroness de Linden.
Dowager Lady Garvagh.
Lady Elizabeth Home.
Lady Leucha Warner.
Lady Eleanor Harbord
Lady Florence Duncombe.
Lady Henrietta Pelham.
Lady Eva Wellesley.
Lady Algernon Percy.
Lady Aline Beaumont.
Lady Blanche Hozier.
Lady Frances Hawke.

Lady Alfred Paget.
Lady Campbell of Garscube.
Lady Erskine.
Lady Mostyn.
Lady Clavering.
Lady Borthwick.
Lady Annesley.
Lady Churchill.
Lady Cavendish.
Lady Wellesley.
The Lady Mayoress (Lady Isaacs).
Mrs. S. B. Bancroft.
Mrs. Bernard Beere.
Miss Ellen Terry.
Mrs. W. H. Kendal.

Earl Cadogan.
Earl of Leitrim.
Lord Rossmore.
Lord Montagu.
Lord Fitz Gerald.
Rt. Hon. Sir John Saville Lumley, Bart.
Sir John Whittaker Ellis, Bart., M.P.
Sir Digby Murray, Bart.
Sir Barnes Peacock, Bart.

Sir Edward Colebrooke. Bart.
Sir Edward Birkbeck, Bart.
Sir Robert Cunliffe, Bart.
Dr. Russell Reynolds, F.R.S., Physician to Her Majesty the Queen's Household.
Sir John Banks, M.D., K.C.B., Physician to Her Majesty the Queen.
Henry Irving, Esq.
Leopold de Rothschild, Esq.

New American Remedy.

A handbill, c. 1890. (Courtesy Wellcome Institute Library, London.)

FOR THE CURE OF COUGHS, COLDS,

CONSUMPTION, ASTHMAS, &c.

LOTT'S
LUNG PILLS

have justly obtained the unqualified approbation of all those who have tried them for speedily curing the Influenza and Bronchitis; also as a most valuable and efficacious Remedy for Colds, Catarrhs, Coughs, Hoarseness, Difficulty of Breathing, Asthma, Consumption, Spitting of Blood, and all disorders of the Lungs. In violent and distressing Coughs they never fail to afford immediate relief, by allaying the tickling and irritation of the Throat and Windpipe, which is the cause of frequent Coughing. They promote Expectoration, remove Fever, Lassitude, and Chilliness. Public Orators and the most Celebrated Vocalists have long held them in the highest estimation for their invaluable properties in removing Huskiness, Wheezing, and Oppression of the Chest, Strengthening the Lungs, and giving Power, Tone, and Clearness to the Voice. A Dose at bed-time seldom fails to cure a recent Cold, and procure sound and refreshing Sleep.

Sold by Appointment of the Proprietor, by

J. W. STIRLING, CHEMIST,

86, HIGH STREET, WHITECHAPEL,

From whom a **SINGLE DOSE** can be had; or in Stamped Boxes at 13½d., 2s. 9d., 4s. 6d. & 11s. each.

(Courtesy Wellcome Institute Library, London.)

Removal of Stones from the Head

A curious form of quackery which prevailed in the seventeenth century and which was taken as a subject for painting by several

Dutch artists (the illustration here is a seventeeth-century drawing on parchment by Pieter Jansz Quast of Amsterdam). It consisted of treating headache or supposed brain disease by extracting a stone from the head. An incision was made in the scalp and the quack took out a stone which he had ready for the purpose—and the patient was cured!

(Courtesy Wellcome Institute Library, London.)

REFERENCE
Br. Med. J. 1911 **1** 1262

A Yorkshire Water Doctor

In the town of Leeds in Yorkshire, there once lived a quack who had received no professional instruction whatever, but was known far and wide for his wonderful cures, and especially for his power of diagnosing the diseases of patients whom he had never seen by simply examining their urine. A celebrated surgeon, Mr X, wishing to see his method of working, desired to be present one day, and the quack readily acceded to his request, feeling much flattered that so great a

The Sick Lady *by Caspar Netscher. (Courtesy Mansell Collection.)*

man should patronise him. Shortly after Mr X had taken his seat a
woman came in with a bottle of urine, which she handed to the quack.
He looked at her, then at the bottle, held it up between him and the
light, shook it, and said 'Your husband's?'.

'Yes, Sir'.

'He is a good deal older than you?'.

'Yes, Sir'.

'He is a tailor?'.

'Yes, Sir'.

'Here' he said, handing her a box of pills, 'tell him to take one of
these pills every night and a big drink of water every morning and he
will soon be all right'.

No sooner had the woman gone out than Mr X turned to the quack,
curious to know how he had made all this out.

'Well, you see', said the quack, 'she was a young woman, and looked well and strong, and I guessed that the water was not hers. I saw she had a wedding ring on her finger so I knew she was married, and I thought that the chances were that it was her husband's water. If he had been about the same age as she it was hardly likely that he was going to be ill either, so I guessed he was older. I knew he was a tailor because the bottle was stopped not with a cork but with a bit of paper rolled up and tied round with a thread in a way no one but a tailor could have done it. Tailors get no exercise and consequently they are all very apt to be constipated. I was quite sure that he would be no exception to the rule and so I gave him opening pills'.

'But how did you know that she came from S?'

'Oh, Mr X have you lived so long in Leeds and don't know the colour of S clay? It was the first thing I saw on her boots the moment she came in'.

REFERENCE
Br. Med. J. 1911 **1** 1261

Eleven Blue Men

This story by Berton Roueché is taken from *The Medical Detectives* (Times Books). It was originally published in the *New Yorker*.

At about eight o'clock on Monday morning, September 25, 1944, a ragged, aimless old man of eighty-two collapsed on the sidewalk on Dey Street, near the Hudson Terminal. Innumerable people must have noticed him, but he lay there alone for several minutes, dazed, doubled up with abdominal cramps, and in an agony of retching. Then a policeman came along. Until the policeman bent over the old man, he may have supposed that he had just a sick drunk on his hands; wanderers dropped by drink are common in that part of town in the early morning. It was not an opinion that he could have held for long. The old man's nose, lips, ears, and fingers were sky-blue. The policeman went to a telephone and put in an ambulance call to Beekman-Downtown Hospital, half a dozen blocks away. The old man was carried into the emergency room there at eight-thirty. By that time, he was unconscious and the blueness had spread over a large part of his body. The examining physician attributed the old man's morbid colour to cyanosis, a condition that usually results from an insufficient supply of oxygen in the blood, and also noted that he was diarrheic and in a severe state of shock. The course of treatment prescribed by the doctor was conventional. It included an instant gastric lavage, heart stimulants, bed rest, and oxygen therapy. Presently, the old man recovered an encouraging, if painful, consciousness and demanded, irascibly and in the name of God, to know what had happened to him. It was a question that, at the moment, nobody could answer with much confidence.

For the immediate record, the doctor made a free-hand diagnosis of carbon-monoxide poisoning—from what source, whether an automobile or a gas pipe, it was, of course, pointless to guess. Then, because an isolated instance of gas poisoning is something of a rarity in a section of the city as crammed with human beings as downtown Manhattan, he and his colleages in the emergency room braced themselves for at least a couple more victims. Their foresight was promptly and generously rewarded. A second man was rolled in at ten-twenty-five. Forty minutes later, an ambulance drove up with three more men. At eleven-twenty, two others were brought in. An additional two arrived during the next fifteen minutes. Around noon, still another was admitted. All of these nine men were also elderly and dilapidated, all had been in misery for at least an hour, and all were rigid, cyanotic, and in a state of shock. The entire body of one, a bony, seventy-three-year-old consumptive named John Mitchell, was blue. Five of the nine, including Mitchell, had been stricken in the Globe Hotel, a sunless, upstairs flophouse at 190 Park Row, and two in a similar place, called the Star Hotel at 3 James Street. Another had been found slumped in the doorway of a condemned building on Park Row, not far from City Hall Park, by a policeman. The ninth had keeled over in front of the Eclipse Cafeteria, at 6 Chatham Square. At a quarter-to-seven that evening, one more aged blue man was brought in. He had been lying, too sick to ask for help, on his cot in a cubicle in the Lion Hotel, another flophouse, at 26 Bowery, since ten o'clock that morning. A clerk had finally looked in and seen him.

By the time this last blue man arrived at the hospital, an investigation of the case by the Department of Health to which all outbreaks of an epidemiological nature must be reported, had been under way for five hours. Its findings thus far had not been illuminating. The investigation was conducted by two men. One was the Health Department's chief epidemiologist, Dr Morris Greenberg, a small, fragile, reflective man of fifty-seven, who is now acting director of the Bureau of Preventable Diseases; the other was Dr Ottavio Pellitteri, a field epidemiologist, who, since 1946, has been administrative medical inspector for the Bureau. He is thirty-six years old, pale, and stocky, and has a bristling black moustache. One day, when I was in Dr Greenberg's office, he and Dr Pellitteri told me about the case. Their recollection of it is, understandably, vivid. The derelicts were the

74

victims of a type of poisoning so rare that only ten previous outbreaks of it had been recorded in medical literature. Of these, two were in the United States and two in Germany; the others had been reported in France, England, Switzerland, Algeria, Australia, and India. Up to September 25, 1944, the largest number of people stricken in a single outbreak was four. That was in Algeria, in 1926.

The Beekman-Downtown Hospital telephoned a report of the occurrence to the Health Department just before noon. As is customary, copies of the report were sent to all the Department's administrative officers. 'Mine was on my desk when I got back from lunch,' Dr Greenberg said to me. 'It didn't sound like much. Nine persons believed to be suffering from carbon-monoxide poisoning had been admitted during the morning, and all of them said they had eaten breakfast at the Eclipse Cafeteria, at 6 Chatham Square. Still, it was a job for us. I checked with the clerk who handles assignments and found that Pellitteri had gone out on it. That was all I wanted to know. If it amounted to anything, I knew he'd phone me before making a written report. That's an arrangement we have here. Well, a couple of hours later I got a call from him. My interest perked right up.'

'I was at the hospital,' Dr Pellitteri told me, 'and I'd talked to the staff and most of the men. There were ten of them by then, of course. They were sick as dogs, but only one was in really bad shape.'

'That was John Mitchell,' Dr Greenberg put in. 'He died the next night. I understand his condition was hopeless from the start. The others, including the old boy who came in last, pulled through all right. Excuse me, Ottavio, but I just thought I'd get that out of the way. Go on.'

Dr Pellitteri nodded. 'I wasn't at all convinced that it was gas poisoning,' he continued. 'The staff was beginning to doubt it, too. The symptoms weren't quite right. There didn't seem to be any of the headache and general dopiness that you get with gas. What really made me suspicious was this: Only two or three of the men had eaten breakfast in the cafeteria at the same time. They had straggled in all the way from seven o'clock to ten. That meant that the place would have had to be full of gas for at least three hours, which is preposterous. It also indicated that we ought to have had a lot more sick people than we did. Those Chatham Square eating places have a big turnover. Well, to make sure, I checked with Bellevue, Gouverneur, St. Vincent's and the other downtown hospitals. None of them had seen a trace of cyanosis. Then I talked to the sick men some more. I learned two interesting things. One was that they had all got sick right after eating. Within thirty minutes. The other was that all but one had eaten oatmeal, rolls, and coffee. He ate just oatmeal. When ten men eat the same thing in the same place on the same day and then all come down with the same illness . . . I told Greenberg that my hunch was food poisoning.'

'I was willing to rule out gas,' Dr Greenberg said. A folder containing data on the case lay on the desk before him. He lifted the cover thoughtfully, then let it drop. 'And I agreed that the oatmeal sounded pretty suspicious. That was as far as I was willing to go. Common, ordinary, everyday food poisoning—I gathered that was what Pellitteri had in mind—wasn't a very satisfying answer. For one thing, cyanosis is hardly symptomatic of that. On the other hand, diarrhoea and severe vomiting are, almost invariably. But they weren't in the clinical picture, I found, except in two or three of the cases. Moreover, the incubation periods—the time lapse between eating and illness—were extremely short. As you probably know, most food poisoning is caused by eating something that has been contaminated by bacteria. The usual offenders are the staphylococci—they're mostly responsible for boils and skin infections and so on—and the salmonella. The latter are related to the typhoid organism. In a staphylococcus case, the first symptoms rarely develop in under two hours. Often, it's closer to five. The incubation period in the other ranges from twelve to thirty-six hours. But here we were with something that hit in thirty minutes or less. Why, one of the men had got only as far as the sidewalk in front of the cafeteria before he was knocked out. Another fact that Pellitteri had dug up struck me as very significant. All of the men told him that the illness had come on with extraordinary suddenness. One minute they were feeling fine, and the next minute they were practically helpless. That was another point against the ordinary food-poisoning theory. Its onset is never that fast. Well, that suddenness began to look like a lead. It led me to suspect that some drug might be to blame. A quick and sudden reaction is characteristic of a great many drugs. So is the combination of cyanosis and shock.'

'None of the men were on dope,' Dr Pellitteri said. 'I told Greenberg I was sure of that. Their pleasure was booze.'

'That was OK,' Dr Greenberg said. 'They could have got a toxic dose of some drug by accident. In the oatmeal, most likely. I couldn't help thinking that the oatmeal was relevant to our problem. At any rate, the drug idea was very persuasive.'

'So was Greenberg,' Dr Pellitteri remarked with a smile. 'Actually, it was the only explanation in sight that seemed to account for everything we knew about the clinical and environmental picture.'

'All we had to do now was prove it,' Dr Greenberg went on mildly. 'I asked Pellitteri to get a blood sample from each of the men before leaving the hospital for a look at the cafeteria. We agreed he would send the specimens to the city toxicologist, Dr Alexander O. Gettler, for an overnight analysis. I wanted to know if the blood contained methemoglobin. Methemoglobin is a compound that's formed only when any one of several drugs enters the blood. Gettler's report would tell us if we were at least on the right track. That is, it would give us a yes-or-no answer on drugs. If the answer was yes, then we could go on from there to identify the particular drug. How we could go about that would depend on what Pellitteri was able to turn up at the cafeteria. In the meantime, there was nothing for me to do but wait for their reports. I'd theorized myself hoarse.'

Dr Pellitteri, having attended to his bloodletting with reasonable dispatch, reached the Eclipse Cafeteria at around five o'clock. 'It was about what I'd expected,' he told me. 'Strictly a horse market, and dirtier than most. The sort of place where you can get a full meal for fifteen cents. There was a grind house on one side, a cigar store on the other, and the 'L' overhead. Incidentally, the Eclipse went out of business a year or so after I was there, but that had nothing to do with us. It was just a coincidence. Well, the place looked deserted and the door was locked. I knocked, and a man came out of the back and let me in. He was one of our people, a health inspector for the Bureau of Food and Drugs, named Weinberg. His bureau had stepped into the case as a matter of routine, because of the reference to a restaurant in the notification report. I was glad to see him and to have his help. For one thing, he had put a temporary embargo on everything in the cafeteria. That's why it was closed up. His main job, though, was to check the place for violations of the sanitation code. He was finding plenty.'

'Let me read you a few of Weinberg's findings,' Dr Greenberg said, extracting a paper from the folder on his desk. 'None of them had any direct bearing on our problem, but I think they'll give you a good idea of what the Eclipse was like—what too many restaurants are like. This copy of his report lists fifteen specific violations. Here they are: "Premises heavily infested with roaches. Fly infestation throughout premises. Floor defective in rear part of dining room. Kitchen walls and ceiling encrusted with grease and soot. Kitchen floor encrusted with dirt. Refuse under kitchen fixtures. Sterilizing facilities inadequate. Sink defective. Floor and walls at serving tables and coffee urns encrusted with dirt. Kitchen utensils encrusted with dirt and grease. Storage-cellar walls, ceiling, and floor encrusted with dirt. Floor and shelves in cellar covered with refuse and useless material. Cellar ceiling defective. Sewer pipe leaking. Open sewer line in cellar." Well . . .' He gave me a squeamish smile and stuck the paper back in the folder.

'I can see it now,' Dr Pellitteri said. 'And smell it. Especially the kitchen, where I spent most of my time. Weinberg had the proprietor and the cook out there, and I talked to them while he prowled around. They were very co-operative. Naturally. They were scared to death. They knew nothing about gas in the place and there was no sign of any, so I went to work on the food. None of what had been prepared for breakfast that morning was left. That, of course, would have been too much to hope for. But I was able to get together some of the kind of stuff that had gone into the men's breakfast, so that we could make a chemical determination at the Department. What I took was ground coffee, sugar, a mixture of evaporated milk and water that passed for cream, some bakery rolls, a five-pound carton of dry oatmeal, and some salt. The salt had been used in preparing the oatmeal. That morning, like every morning, the cook told me, he had prepared six gallons of oatmeal, enough to serve around a hundred and twenty-five people. To make it, he used five pounds of dry cereal, four gallons of water—regular city water—and a handful of salt. That was his term—a handful. There was an open gallon can of salt standing on the stove. He said the handful he'd put in that morning's otameal had come from that. He refilled the can on the stove every morning from a big supply can. He pointed out the big can—it was up on a shelf—and as I was getting it down to take with me, I saw another can, just like it, nearby. I took that one down, too. It was also full of salt, or, rather, something that looked like salt. The proprietor said it wasn't salt. He said it was saltpetre—sodium nitrate—that he used in corning beef and in making pastrami. Well, there isn't any harm in saltpetre; it doesn't even act as an anti-aphrodisiac, as a lot of people seem to think. But I wrapped it up with the other loot and took it along, just for fun. The fact is, I guess, everything in that damn place looked like poison.'

After Dr Pellitteri had deposited his loot with a Health Department chemist, Andrew J. Pensa, who promised to have a report ready by the following afternoon, he dined hurriedly at a restaurant in which he had confidence and returned to Chatham Square. There he spent the evening making the rounds of the lodging houses in the neighbourhood. He had heard at Mr Pensa's office that an eleventh blue man had been admitted to the hospital, and before going home he wanted to make sure that no other victims had been overlooked. By midnight, having covered all the likely places and having rechecked the downtown hospitals, he was satisfied. He repaired to his office and composed a formal progress report for Dr Greenberg. Then he went home and to bed.

The next morning, Tuesday, Dr Pellitteri dropped by the Eclipse, which was still closed but whose proprietor and staff he had told to return for questioning. Dr Pellitteri had another talk with the proprietor and the cook. He also had a few inconclusive words with the rest of the cafeteria's employees—two dishwashers, a busboy, and a counterman. As he was leaving, the cook, who had apparently passed an uneasy night with his conscience, remarked that it was possible that he had absent-mindedly refilled the salt can on the stove from the one that contained saltpetre. 'That was interesting,' Dr Pellitteri told me, 'even though such a possibility had already occurred to me, and even though I didn't know whether it was important or not. I assured him that he had nothing to worry about. We had been certain all along that nobody had deliberately poisoned the old men.' From the Eclipse, Dr Pellitteri went on to Dr Greenberg's office, where Dr Gettler's report was waiting.

'Gettler's test for methemoglobin was positive,' Dr Greenberg said. 'It had to be a drug now. Well, so far so good. Then we heard from Pensa.'

'Greenberg almost fell out of his chair when he read Pensa's report,' Dr Pellitteri observed cheerfully.

'That's an exaggeration,' Dr Greenberg said. 'I'm not easily dumbfounded. We're inured to the incredible around here. Why, a few years ago we had a case involving some numbskull who stuck a fistful of potassium-thiocyanate crystals, a very nasty poison, in the coils of an office water cooler, just for a practical joke. However, I can't deny that Pensa rather taxed our credulity. What he had found was that the small salt can and the one that was supposed to be full of sodium nitrate both contained sodium nitrite. The other food samples, incidentally, were OK.'

'That also taxed my credulity,' Dr Pellitteri said.

Dr. Greenberg smiled. 'There's a great deal of difference between nitrate and nitrite,' he continued. 'Their only similarity, which is an unfortunate one, is that they both look and taste more or less like ordinary table salt. Sodium nitrite isn't the most powerful poison in the world, but a little of it will do a lot of harm. If you remember, I said before that this case was almost without precedent—only ten outbreaks like it on record. Ten is practically none. In fact, sodium-nitrite poisoning is so unusual that some of the standard texts on toxicology don't even mention it. So Pensa's report was pretty startling. But we accepted it, of course, without question or hesitation. Facts are facts. And we were glad to. It seemed to explain everything very nicely. What I've been saying about sodium-nitrite poisoning doesn't mean that sodium nitrite itself is rare. Actually, it's fairly common. It's used in the manufacture of dyes and as a medical drug. We use it in treating certain heart conditions and for high blood pressure. But it also has another important use, one that made its presence at the Eclipse sound plausible. In recent years, and particularly during the war, sodium nitrite has been used as a substitute for sodium nitrate in preserving meat. The government permits it but stipulates that the finished meat must not contain more than one part of sodium nitrite per five thousand parts of meat. Cooking will safely destroy enough of that small quantity of the drug.' Dr Greenberg shrugged. 'Well, Pellitteri had had the cook pick up a handful of salt—the same amount, as nearly as possible, as went into the oatmeal—and then had taken this to his office and found that it weighed approximately a hundred grams. So we didn't have to think twice to realize that the proportion of nitrite in that batch of cereal was considerably higher than one to five thousand. Roughly, it must have been around one to about eighty before cooking destroyed part of the nitrite. It certainly looked as though Gettler, Pensa, and the cafeteria cook between them had given us our answer. I called up Gettler and told him what Pensa had discovered and asked him to run a specific test for nitrites on his blood samples. He had, as a matter of course, held some blood back for later examination. His confirmation came through in a couple of hours. I went home that night feeling pretty good.'

Dr Greenberg's serenity was a fugitive one. He awoke on Wednesday morning troubled in mind. A question had occurred to him that he was unable to ignore. 'Something like a hundred and twenty-five people ate oatmeal at the Eclipse that morning,' he said to me, 'but only eleven of them got sick. Why? The undeniable fact that those eleven old men were made sick by the ingestion of a toxic dose of sodium nitrite wasn't enough to rest on. I wanted to know exactly how much sodium nitrite each portion of that cooked oatmeal had contained. With Pensa's help again, I found out. We prepared a batch just like the one the cook had made on Monday. Then Pensa measured out six ounces, the size of the average portion served at the Eclipse, and analyzed it. It contained two and a half grams of sodium nitrite. That explained why the hundred and fourteen other people did not become ill. The toxic dose of sodium nitrite is three grains. But it didn't explain how each of our eleven old men had received an additional half grain. It seemed extremely unlikely that the extra touch of nitrite had been in the oatmeal when it was served. It had to come in later. Then I began to get a glimmer. Some people sprinkle a little salt, instead of sugar, on hot cereal. Suppose, I thought, that the busboy, or whoever had the job of keeping the table salt shakers filled, had made the same mistake that the cook had. It seemed plausible. Pellitteri was out of the office—I've forgotten where—so I got Food and Drugs to step over to the Eclipse, which was still under embargo, and bring back the shakers for Pensa to work on. There were seventeen of them, all good-sized, one for each table. Sixteen contained either pure sodium chloride or just a few inconsequential traces of sodium nitrite mixed in with the real salt, but the other was point thirty-seven per cent nitrite. That one was enough. A spoonful of that salt contained a bit more than half a grain.'

'I went over to the hospital Thursday morning,' Dr Pellitteri said. 'Greenberg wanted me to check the table-salt angle with the men. They could tie the case up neatly for us. I drew a blank. They'd been discharged the night before, and God only knew where they were.'

'Naturally,' Dr Greenberg said, 'It would have been nice to know for a fact that the old boys all sat at a certain table and that all of them put about a spoonful of salt from that particular shaker on their oatmeal, but it wasn't essential. I was morally certain that they had. There just wasn't any other explanation. There was one other question, however. Why did they use so *much* salt? For my own peace of mind, I wanted to know. All of a sudden, I remembered Pellitteri had said they were all heavy drinkers. Well, several recent clinical studies have demonstrated that there is usually a subnormal concentration of sodium chloride in the blood of alcoholics. Either they don't eat enough to get sufficient salt or they lose it more rapidly than other people do, or both. Whatever the reasons are, the conclusion was all I needed. Any animal, you know, whether a mouse or a man, tends to try to obtain a necessary substance that his body lacks. The final question had been answered.'

© Berton Roueché 1948.

Old Dog, New Tricks

Contributed by Monica Harding (who was the lady from Liverpool) and extracted from *World Medicine* 11 February 1976, p. 102.

A lady from Liverpool related how something rather bizarre happened when she took the occupants of an old folk's home on a river cruise. Down in the loo, an octogenarian lady called Mildred suddenly decided she needed a tampon and put a coin in the machine . . . which promptly stuck.

Spellbound at the thought of medical history in the making, my correspondent handed her another coin; out popped the object in question. The old lady heaved a sigh of relief and gasped:

'Thanks, luv. I'm dying for a fag.'
Her friend, slightly older, interposed:

'They're not ciggies, Mildred. They're sweets—and you're on a diet so give them to me.'

Alas, history does not record the effect of this unusual confection on her gastrointestinal tract!

A Barber Surgeon Operating in His Office

The plate with the indented rim, resting on the window ledge to the right, was held under the chin of his customers while he shaved them. The stuffed animal suspended from the ceiling was intended to keep away evil spirits. A stuffed alligator was usually sufficient for this purpose.

REFERENCE
Haggard H W 1929 *Devils, Dugs and Doctors* (London: Heinemann)

The Indian Manner of Blood-letting

A Central American native letting the blood by piercing the patient's arm with an arrow. From 'The new voyage and description of the isthmus of America' by Lionel Wafer, published in London, 1699. The illustration relates to Panama in 1681.

Breathing a Vein

1804 engraving by H Humphrey, London. (Courtesy Wellcome Institute Library, London.)

Rejects

The Chinese are certainly a sweet and sour lot. An English writer has just received quite the most elegant letter of rejection, from a Chinese economics magazine: 'We have read your manuscript with boundless delight. If we were to publish your paper, it would be impossible for us to publish any work of a lower standard;

'And as it is unthinkable that, in the next 1000 years we shall see its equal, we are, to our regret, compelled to return your divine composition and beg you a 1000 times to overlook our short sight and timidity.' Oh well, all right, since you put it like that.

REFERENCE
Observer 25 September 1983

Setting Limbs

Illustration from a thirteenth-century treatise on surgery which was translated from the Latin of Roger of Salerno. (Courtesy Mansell Collection.)

Physician's Tombstone

The carving of a doctor about to make his diagnosis is from the family tomb of the famous Greek physician, Jason. (Courtesy Mansell Collection.)

French Proverb

Forty is the old age of youth but fifty is the youth of old age.

Consultation with a Thirteenth-century Arab Physician

Medical learning was highly developed in all the chief cities of Moslem power, and in the eleventh century Arabian medicine began to be

(Courtesy Mansell Collection.)

(Courtesy Mansell Collection.)

known through translations in the western world. For example, in Sicily it was encouraged by King Frederick II, who as a youth had several Saracen teachers.

The two pictures are from fragments of an Arabic translation, dated 1222, of the *Materia Medica* of Dioscorides, a Greek physician who lived *c*. 90–40 BC. One of the Arabic paintings is of a consultation between doctor and patient whereas the other is of a clinical consultation involving several doctors.

The Earliest Recorded Clinical Trial

Nebuchadnezzar II, having invested Jerusalem and defeated the Israelis in 600 BC, took several youths back to his own country for indoctrination and training. They were carefully selected. All were of royal or princely blood, social class 1 in fact. All were physically fit with a high IQ. They were to be put on a rigid diet of meat and wine for three years with one of the eunuchs acting as the monitor. Daniel persuaded the monitor to give him and three others a diet of pulse and water for ten days, when, it is recorded, they were fairer in countenance and fatter in body than the other subjects who were given meat and wine. Daniel had ruined the trial, the eunuch had defied the King, and the trial had become uncontrolled. It was not recorded what Nebuchadnezzar did to the eunuch.

REFERENCE
Book of Daniel ch. 1

Malingering

In the following article, Richard Asher[1,2] has provided what is probably the best published essay on malingering:

I do not want my contribution to consist only of anecdotes about malingerers, so I shall not spend long recounting stories of ingenious patients who fooled the doctors or tales of clever doctors and how they caught the patient in the act.

The pride of a doctor who has caught a malingerer is akin to that of a fisherman who has landed an enormous fish; and his stories (like those of fisherman) may become somewhat exaggerated in the telling.

Nor will I spend long on the details of technique: where the pins were hidden, how the blood was obtained, how the food was disposed of and how the thermometer was manipulated. These are matters of prestidigitation and are more worthy of consideration by the Magic Circle than by the Medical Society of London.

I am not going to confine myself to pure malingering, but I shall also discuss the borderland of malingering which provides even more difficult and obscure cases for study.

True malingering is defined in the *Concise Oxford Dictionary* as the pretending production or protraction of illness in order to escape duty, especially in soldiers and sailors. I allow a wider meaning to the term. To start with, I do not exclude the Air Force, especially as I remember an aircraftsman treated by Squadron Leader Harry Gosset who was a genuine haemophiliac and required over twenty pints of blood to stop the bleeding from his appendicectomy wound. This poor fellow, believing he was dying and wishing to confess his sins, admitted that he had simulated his appendicitis to get home for Christmas. He said he would never have done this had he known there would be so much bleeding trouble.

I define malingering as the imitation, production or encouragement of illness for a deliberate end. The patient is quite conscious of what he is doing and quite cognisant of why he is doing it. With that definition, pure malingering—the planned fraudulent faking of illness —is, in my experience, a very rare condition. Either that, or else I am a very gullible physician. I know I have been mistaken before now and it is possible that many malingerers have deceived me without being suspected. I shall show you the portrait of a case where I was grossly deceived. It was over a matter of malingering associated with hysterical ataxia, scissor gait and aggressive outbursts.

One Sunday, when my daughter was two years old, I promised my wife that, if it was not taken as a precedent, I would myself get her up from her afternoon rest, dress her and take her for a walk. I performed these duties without difficulty or loss of dignity, until the walk started. Then there was trouble. The child kept falling to the left; she walked with a ridiculous scissor gait and she frequently fell to the ground. She cried and said she had a pain. She behaved abominably, and I spent a wretched afternoon in Park Square West attempting to coax her into good behaviour. I knew this was sheer devilment, a malignant aggressive demonstration against the father figure; I would not submit.

At last my wife returned and undressed her for her evening bath. There was a sudden cry:—'Do you realise you've put both her legs through the same hole in her knickers?' I can still remember, after those tortured limbs had been freed from the crippling garments, how that gay, naked figure raced unrestrictedly to the bathroom without a trace of malingering. That incident taught me to be cautious about diagnosing malingering or hysteria. These diagnoses must not be made for the sole reason that the clinical picture is not yet hung in the clinical picture gallery of the doctor in charge. It may be something he hasn't heard of. There are too many examples of apparent malingering turning out to be cases of organic disease, and jokes about the high mortality of malingering or hysteria are commonplace.

I could show you a picture of a lady who had a lesion on her face and other lesions on her fingers and elsewhere. For a long time they were thought to be self inflicted, but biopsy studies have left no doubt that she is suffering from Phagaedena Geometricum of Von Brocq, and the control of the lesions by cortisone has brought great relief to the patient and to her doctor.

A young National Serviceman, who complained for over a year of peculiar abdominal pains, was thought to be malingering, but in the end he was found to have Von Recklinghausen's neurofibromatosis of the intestine, and several members of his family were discovered to be afflicted by the same rare condition.

Nevertheless, genuine authenticated malingering does occur. True malingering is best classified by motives rather than by techniques—- the principal prime movers being Fear, Desire and Escape.

Fear: fear of call-up, fear of overseas duty, fear of warfare.

Desire: desire for compensation, desire for a comfortable pension, desire for revenge against a surgeon for some (usually imagined) wrong. Desire for the comforts of hospital life. Desire to stay in the ward longer because one has fallen in love with the staff nurse.

Escape: escape from a prisoner-of-war camp by uncurable disability, escape from prison by transfer to hospital, escape from an impending court case, escape from battle.

Malingering by prisoners of war has evolved a variety of ingenious techniques, even to the extent of passing borrowed albuminuric urine, secreted in a false bladder and passed in the presence of a suspicious German doctor, through a hand-carved and hand-painted penis of life-like verisimilitude. The technical term for such realistic art is *trompe l'oeil,* an expression usually applied to oil painting but presumably correct for sculpture and wood carving.

It is well known that opposing forces try to weaken the enemy's army by dropping pamphlets persuading them to malinger. A particular pamphlet dropped in large numbers early in 1945 on English troops in Italy is worthy of your attention. Neatly produced in book-match form (to make it easy to hide), it opens with Three Golden Rules for Malingering which I do not think could be beaten:

90

1. You must make the impression you hate to be ill.
2. Make up your mind for one disease and stick to it.
3. Don't tell the doctor too much.

This pamphlet catered for all tastes and resembles the 'Do it Yourself' guides so popular today.

There is only time to give details about one of those. Here is how to have tuberculosis—according to the instruction book:

'First you must smoke excessively to acquire a cough. Then tell the doctor that you have lost weight, you do not feel well and that you cough a great deal. Say that sometimes you cough up streaks of blood. Sometimes you wake drenched with sweat. Stick to these symptoms, do not invent any new ones.

'Mix a very little blood with your sputum; suck it from your gums or a prick on your finger, one or two drops are sufficient.' Then there follow certain supplementary techniques of which I propose to omit the details. They concern the correct use of the smegma bacillus to enrich the bacteriology of the sputum. They are not attractive. The instructions finish with these encouraging words: 'All the above directions are based on scientific observations in well-known University Hospitals.'

The pamphlet was printed in the *Lancet* who gave it rather a discouraging review as follows: The authors would be disappointed to see how lightly their elaborate propaganda is received by our soldiers. They say they know far better tricks than these!

At Cardiff last week an ex-prisoner-of-war, Dr Archie Cochrane, told me a technique (he called it 'Fudging' X-rays) whereby he annually returned three healthy prisoners to England totally disabled with radiological tuberculosis.

Painting in barium requires delicate brushwork very different from painting in oils. The technique of Van Gogh is useless for painting tuberculosis cavities however suitable it may be for sunflowers.

The general run of malingerers are of poor intelligence, and naivety rather than ingenuity is the rule. Among ingenious and distinguished malingerers Sherlock Holmes is worth recalling. In 'The Case of the Dying Detective' Holmes had to convince Watson that he was dying of an obscure tropical disease. He started by reducing Watson's limited faculties to their lowest ebb:

'Facts are facts, Watson. You are only a general practitioner with very limited experience and mediocre qualifications. It is painful for me to have to say these things but you give me no choice. Shall I demonstrate your own ignorance?

'What do you know, pray, of Tapanuli Fever? What do you know of the Black Formosa Corruption?'

Mr. President, I do not wish to discomfort you in front of this distinguished audience, but can you improve on Watson's answer: 'I have never heard of either'?

After this preliminary humiliation Holmes had little difficulty in convincing Watson, who in his turn convinced the villain—Culverton Smith—that he, Holmes, was dying. At the end of the case when Culverton Smith was in handcuffs and Holmes had revived himself with claret and biscuits, he described his methods: Three days of fast does not improve one's beauty. Then, with Vaseline upon one's forehead, belladonna in one's eyes, rouge over the cheek-bones and crusts of beeswax round one's lips, a very satisfying effect can be produced. A little occasional talk about half-crowns, oysters, or any other extraneous subjects produces a pleasing effect of delirium.

Mention of the imitation of delirium reminds one that mental as well as physical disease can be simulated. Those with little experience of mental disease may learn with surprise that it is very hard to pretend to be mad. For instance, the peculiar distorted thinking of the schizophrenic is something a sane person cannot manage. An experiment was done in which twenty normal people were asked to feign insanity; they, and twenty genuinely psychotic patients, were interviewed by psychiatrists (who had no other means of telling which was which). The psychiatrists were able to pick out the malingerers in nearly ninety per cent of the cases. Yet the most remarkable feat of feigning insanity was carried out by Lieut. Jones and Lieut. Hill who were prisoners in Yozgad, Turkey, in 1917. They were carefully coached by a fellow-prisoner who was a doctor and they went through almost unendurable privations in their successful pretence of madness. Their book, *The Road to Endor*, is still a best seller and a classic.

I now pass to those cases of illness which, though self produced or prolonged, do not constitute malingering. They do not have so definite a purpose. As you see, I have grouped them together as The Borderland of Malingering.

The Advantages of Illness

1. Illness as a Purpose (True Malingering)
2. Illness as a Comfort (Hysteria)
3. Illness as a Hobby (Hypochondriasis)
4. Illness as a Profession (Psychopaths)

The Borderland of Malingering

Hysterics differ from malingerers because, although they may produce illness and enjoy it, they are unaware of what they are doing. They possess a capacity for self-deception; they can wall off part of their mind so that it is impervious to self scrutiny. This process, dignified by psychiatrists with the term 'dissociation', is colloquially called 'kidding yourself'. Some cases of hysteria are very close to malingering. Others start as malingerers, and as they become better at kidding

92

others, they finally succeed in kidding themselves, and become hysterics.

The Borderland of Malingering

A. Illness as a comfort
- (*a*) Hysteria.
- (*b*) The Proud Lonely Person (Lucy's disease).

B. *Illness as a hobby*
- (*a*) The Grand Tour Type (rich hypochondriac).
- (*b*) The Chronic Out-Patient (poor hypochondriac).
- (*c*) The Eccentric Hypochondriac (faddist).
- (*d*) The Chronic Convalescent (daren't recover).

C. Illness as a profession
- (*a*) Anorexia Nervosa.
- (*b*) The Chronic Artefactualists.
- (*c*) Munchausen's Syndrome.

I have seen very little proven hysteria and I diagnose the condition only with diffidence. A fair proportion of 'hysterics' turn out to have organic disease, as many of us know to our cost.

Notice that among illness as a comfort I have put the proud, lonely person. Allow me to explain this. This pathetic type of case usually occurs in later life when praise and companionship are hard to come by. To lonely people a medical consultation may represent an event of great importance. It supplies that need to be noticed that exists in all human beings. A child cries: 'Look at my sandcastle!' A lonely old person cries: 'Look at my stomach.' The child says: 'I got two goals this afternoon!' The lonely old person says: 'I got two giddy turns this afternoon.'

I have heard from more than one practitioner of elderly people who have a weekly or fortnightly consultation of this kind. A visit from the doctor allows them the illusion of seeking medical advice rather than companionship. A patient may be too proud to complain of loneliness, but there is no loss of pride in complaining of symptoms. Lonely people miss, not only companionship, but also the advice and criticism that go with it. Under the guise of seeking advice about health, a lonely lady may be seeking advice about family affairs. Ostensibly she is asking for advice about her bad heart, but *au fond* she seeks advice about her bad nephew. This mild and most benign form of malingering, in which solitary elderly people look for company or counsel under the thin disguise of chronic ill health, is understandably tolerated or even enjoyed by quite a lot of practitioners. It could well be called Lucy's disease after Wordsworth's Lucy:

> She dwelt among the untrodden ways
> Beside the springs of Dove,
> A maid whom there were none to praise
> And very few to love.

Turning to the hypochondriacs, first we have the rich hypochondriac. I call this one The Grand Tour Type, because she spends much of her time touring the larger cities in Europe visiting consultants. She always carries a large dossier, opinions from consultants, X-rays and laboratory reports; and usually a list of her own symptoms which she has carefully written out. During her tour she may have persuaded surgeons to remove some of her less essential organs. She has usually had her gall bladder and a quota of her pelvic organs removed by the time she reaches one's consulting room. Such women discuss consultants with their friends as one recommends a fashionable tailor or a smart hairdresser, and rival each other in the grandeur of the consultants they have visited as well as in the complexities of their investigations and treatments. They are usually married to rich but unattentive husbands who supply them with money for their hobby as a substitute for affection. To the consultant in private practice they are a familiar, tedious and lucrative burden.

The poor hypochondriac (or perpetual out-patient). Every hospital has a number of out-patients who have attended for many years. Whenever they are discharged from one department they turn up in another, thus acquiring a very large collection of documents, rivalling that of the rich hypochondriac although written on less luxurious writing paper and penned by less illustrious names. Though some have genuine chronic illness, many of them attend because they like the companionship of hospital; instead of going to the local public house for a glass of beer and a chat with the landlord, they go to the hospital for a bottle of medicine and a chat with the other patients. One enlightened doctor tried the experiment of arranging out-patient sessions where the patients did not see the doctor at all unless they asked for him. It was a great success.

The eccentric hypochondriacs. These people like peculiar or unorthodox treatments. They like so-called 'natural' things and belong to the homespun, wholemeal, handicraft school of living. They know a clever little man who can find out what is wrong with you by holding a pendulum over you or using some form of magic box. They believe with apostolic fervour in nature cures, osteopaths, astrologers and herbalists. Their preoccupation is more with treatment than with illness and they are harmless and often entertaining.

The chronic convalescent. When a patient has had longstanding organic disease for many years it becomes so familiar to him that it is almost a friend. If the illness is suddenly cured, he may feel deserted

94

and friendless. He misses the familiar pain, the sympathetic enquiries of his friends and the security of his medical routine. He feels like a man who has worn shoes so long that he can no longer go barefoot. He does not really want to get well; he has become a hypochondriac.

Now the last group: Illness as a profession. First, I consider anorexia nervosa. The reason why these people go to such lengths to avoid eating is rarely clear. They will resort to a variety of artifices to avoid food. They will hide food in their bed lockers, pour milk into their hot-water bottles and insist on starving in the midst of plenty. As a result of the starvation, amenorrhoea is an early symptom and this formerly led to the illness being confused with Simmonds disease, with which it has nothing to do.

The next group is that of the chronic artefactualists, who may spend years in self-mutilation or the production of spurious fevers. Skin diseases are most favoured by the sufferers from chronic autogenous disease, but various other forms of self-damage are reported. A group of nineteen patients was reported by workers in the Psychological Medicine Department of the Birmingham Hospitals under the title 'Deliberate Disability'. Their most surprising finding was that most of these patients are highly intelligent. One possibility is that their intelligence prevents them from learning the art of hysterical dissociation. One young woman was referred to me by Dr Harold Wilson. She was a bit of a problem child; she had been more or less bald for several years and he suspected the condition was due to trichotilomania (dermatologese for hair-pulling). He suggested that hypnosis, which is a part-time activity of mine, might stop her. At our first interview I asked her if it was possible she was occasionally pulling hairs out of her scalp. She said, yes, she thought she was. I then said as it seemed to be making her bald it might be a good idea to stop pulling her hair out. She said, all right, she would try. That was the only treatment given. I never used hypnosis on her at all and yet she had a normal head of hair within three months.

Lastly, Munchausen's syndrome. This is the strangest and rarest form of chronic autogenous disease. I described and named the syndrome in a paper in the *Lancet* seven years ago, but it had been recognised for generations; all I did was to provide a convenient label.

Munchausen's Syndrome
Three main types

A. Laparotomophilia migrans.
   With mainly abdominal symptoms.
B. Haemorrhagica histrionica.
   Colloquially—'haemoptysis merchant,' 'haematemesis merchant.'
   Largely specialising in haemorrhage.
C. Neurologica diabolica.
   Specialising in faints, fits, stupor, etc.

The patient with this syndrome is nearly always brought into hospital by police or bystanders, having collapsed in the street or on a bus with an apparently acute illness, supported by a plausible and yet dramatic history. Though his history seems most convincing at first, later his story is found to be largely false, and his symptoms and signs mostly spurious. He is discovered to have attended and deceived an astounding number of other hospitals. At several of them he may have been operated upon, and a large number of abdominal scars is often found. So skilfully do these people imitate acute illness that the diagnosis may be quite unsuspected until a passing doctor, ward sister or hospital porter says 'I know that man—we had him in St Quinidines last September. He says he's an ex-fighter pilot shot in the chest, in the last war, and he coughs up blood; or sometimes he's been shot through the head in the last war and has fits.'

These people differ from other chronic artefactualists in their constant progression from one hospital to another, often under a variety of false names, but nearly always telling the same story. They rarely stay at one hospital for long, but, if not already ejected, discharge themselves within a few days and off they go on their wanderings, deceiving one hospital after another, telling the same false story, faking the same fictitious symptoms and submitting to innumerable operations and investigations.

Almost all of you have encountered examples of this, but I still say it is rare. It seems common because the afflicted (or afflicting) patients never stop working for a moment. One patient may visit over fifty hospitals in a year. With Munchausen's syndrome a little goes a long way, or, as Churchill might put it: Never in the history of medicine have so many been so much annoyed by so few.

The term Munchausen's syndrome is not beyond criticism and various other names, such as Hospital Hoboes, have been suggested, but the term is convenient and seems to stick.

The gentleman to whom I respectfully dedicated this syndrome originated as a real person—Hieronymus Karl Frederick Von Munchausen of Brunswick—who was wont to entertain his friends by recounting fabulous adventures of palpable absurdity. When Rudloph Raspe of Hanover anonymously published these stories without his permission, a gentlemanly old fellow with a gift for tall stories became the laughing stock of Europe and the eponymous representation of an incorrigible liar. It is to Raspe's fictitious Baron that my term refers; the patients resemble him in the dramatic nature of their stories, the wide extent of their travels and the untruthfulness of their tales.

I must tell you one of Baron Munchausen's stories, for they are truly splendid. The Baron tells how he was out hunting one day and, just when he had used up all his shot, he met a huge stag. In this

96

emergency he charged his gun with cherry stones and let fly, hitting the animal in the forehead. The stag was momentarily stunned, staggered a few paces and made off into the forest. Two years later he was out hunting again when he encountered a particularly noble stag. Luckily on this occasion he was better equipped with ammunition and, after despatching the beast, he lunched off haunch of venison with cherry sauce, for there was a flourishing cherry tree growing from the beast's head.

The stories told by Munchausen patients are equally untrue, but less inherently unlikely; indeed it is the credibility of their stories that makes these patients such a perpetual and tedious problem. It seems that nothing can be done to prevent their continuing clinical depredations. Most doctors are so pleased if they succeed with detection and ejection they never think about protection. Though serious psychiatric studies of these people have been made, nobody can yet answer the two fundamental questions:

(*a*) Why do they do it?
(*b*) How can we stop them doing it?

It is lucky there are so few of them.

All that can be said about them, and indeed about the whole subject of malingering, are these words of Robert Burns:

But human bodies are such fools
For all their colleges and schools
That when no real ills do perplex them
They make enough themselves to vex them.

Shall we leave it at that then? The best explanation for all this self-manufactured disease is simply this: That human beings are such fools.

REFERENCES
[1] Asher R 1958–9 *Trans. Med. Soc.* **75**
[2] Asher R 1972 *Richard Asher Talking Sense* pp 145–55 (London: Pitman Medical). By permission of Pitman Publishing Ltd, London

---

Milk Transfusion

An alternative to blood transfusion was tried in Toronto in 1854 during a cholera epidemic: transfusion of cow's milk. The underlying rationale was that milk would turn into white blood cells. Of the seven patients treated by intravenous transfusion of 12 ounces of milk, five died but two allegedly got better. Twenty years later in New York, intravenous sheep milk infusion was used as a treatment for terminal tuberculosis for two patients. One died in four hours and the other in 24 hours. Seven more patients were treated in New York between 1875 and 1879, by a Dr T G Thomas who claimed that fever, tachycardia and headache were all improved after a while, and predicted a 'brilliant and advantageous future' for intravenous milk infusion. Some enthusiasts even went so far as to predict that milk would eventually replace blood completely in transfusion work.

REFERENCE
Sterpellone L 1986 *Instruments for Health* Farmitalia (Carlo Erba: Freiburg i. Br.) pp 90–2

Cow Pearl Jam

From the Khan el Khalili bazaar, Cairo, 1983.

Some 50 years ago, Egyptian ladies were only considered to be beautiful if they were fat and to enhance this process they were given Cow Pearl jam whose ingredients are given below, together with the Arabic marketing slogan.

COW PEARL JAM

Honey
Aleppo pistachios
Iraqi dates
Carbohydrates (probably flour!)
Shelled almonds
Moroccan sage
Gall-stones from the cow (this is the active ingredient!)

For vivaciousness, beauty and anti-slimming and anti-cachexia for women, men, girls and boys supposed to give you an appetite.

Gin Mania in London

Gin was first developed in 1650 by Franciscus Sylvius, professor of medicine at the State University of Leyden in Holland. To produce a medicine with diuretic properties, he distilled the juniper berry with spirits derived from fermented barley. The French name for juniper, *genièvre*, was the origin of the English name, gin, for the resultant alcoholic refreshment which also became known by the term Mother's Ruin. It was introduced in England early in the eighteenth century by soldiers returning from the Low Countries, and it rapidly become a national addiction. This was not because of its taste, though, but because of vested interests. Beer and ale had been taxed since 1643, but gin was not because its production gave farmers a market for cereal at a time when prices were low and because of the political power of the distillers.

Between 1715 and 1750, gin mania reached epidemic proportions in London, a city which in 1736 contained more than 7000 gin houses, representing one house in every six. During this period it was blamed for the occurrences of more deaths than births in London, with the greatest mortality among children. Burials of those younger than five years represented some three-quarters of all children who had been christened.

It was in London that a strong counter-reaction began to the gin mania, primarily in the arts and letters of the time. This alcoholic way of life and its incongruities were held up for ridicule by writers such as Henry Fielding in his novels *Joseph Andrews* and *The History of Tom Jones*, by composers such as John Gay in *The Beggar's Opera* and by artists such as William Hogarth in engravings. Fielding, who became a magistrate in Westminster, quoted:

99

> What must become of the infant who is conceived in gin with the poisonous distillations of which it is nourished both in the womb and at the breast?

and a statement of the overall problem was made by the Middlesex Sessions Committee in 1735:

> Unhappy mothers habituate themselves to these distilled liquors, whose children are born weak and sickly, and often looked shrivel's and old.

William Hogarth (1697–1764) attacked the social evils of his day with graphic depiction of the reality of London society in the first half of the eighteenth century. One of his most effective and best known satirical engravings is *Gin Lane*, published in 1751. It is one of his many allusions to the detrimental effects of alcohol on society and certainly his most comprehensive and biting. According to Hogarth himself:

> In Gin Lane every circumstance of its horrid effects are brought in view, in teorem nothing but Poverty misery and ruin are to be seen Distress even to madness and death, and not a house in tolerable condition but the Pawnbrokers and the Gin Shop.

The overall impression in *Gin Lane* is that of total disintegration of society through the depiction of general tumult, disorderliness, collapse of buildings, and agitated persons and groups. The period of 1700–50 was a time of severe hardship for the poor in England and of disregard to public health measures. Prostitution and venereal disease were rife. Robbery, brutality and murder were common and hanging was an acceptable punishment for theft of as little as a shilling. These elements of dissipation and callousness were heightened in London and alcohol became almost a necessity for lower-class Londoners of the eighteenth century to tolerate the cold, the abject poverty, the filth and the hopelessness of their environment. Gin, because it was cheap, became the opiate of the massess who spent their meagre income for solace rather than for staple food.

More specific effects of alcohol are depicted in *Gin Lane*. On the left a carpenter is pawning the tools of his trade for gin. In the right upper corner, the suicide by hanging is that of a barber, as indicated by the adjacent barber's pole, In the right lower corner, an emaciated and dying man is still clutching his bottle of gin. The centre background of the engraving is highlighted by the sign of an undertaker, a hanging coffin. Also depicted are several detrimental effects of alcohol on infants of gin addiction. Close to the undertaker's sign, a female body is being lowered into a coffin. Besides the coffin is a neglected infant. To the right of this pitiful tableau is a more macabre event. A mad-

100

Gin Lane by William Hogarth. (Courtesy Wellcome Institute Library, London.)

dened alcoholic has skewered a live child on his staff. A less violent
event, but still child abuse, is in the right central margin of the
engraving. A woman is forcing gin into an unwilling infant. Immediately above this, a consequence is seen in the form of two schoolgirls
who are voluntarily drinking gin. The most dominant figure is in the
foreground of the engraving—an unkempt, stupified woman whose
unattended child is falling to his death. The facial appearance of the
child is worthy of note. The eyes have a shorter than normal palpebral
fissure, resulting in relatively round 'Orphan Annie' eyes. These are
one of the effects of maternal alcohol on fetal morphogenesis as
described in a paper in the *Lancet* of 1973[1].

REFERENCES

Text adapted from Rodin A E 1981 'Infants and gin mania in 18th century
London' *J. Am. Med. Assoc.* **245** 1237–9
[1] Jones K L *et al* 1973 'Pattern of malformation in offspring of chronic
alcoholic mothers' *Lancet* **1** 1267–71

Nicholas Copernicus and the Inception of Bread-Buttering

During the first quarter of the sixteenth century, the small principality of Ermland was the scene of frequent and terrible devastation. It bordered the Gulf of Danzig and was one of four dioceses into which Prussia had been divided for purposes of ecclesiastical government. The bishop of Ermland, Copernicus' uncle, was frequently engaged in conflict with the Order of Teutonic Knights which had formerly ruled Ermland and they periodically launched military expeditions to regain supremacy. There were three fortified towns in the bishopric and one of these was Allenstein, on the River Alle. Copernicus, appointed to the sinecure of canon of Frauenberg Cathedral by his uncle, was also commandant of Allenstein Castle.

The final attempt of the Teutonic Knights to reassert suzerainty occurred between the years 1519 and 1521, and in 1520 they beseiged Allenstein Castle which was considered to be a strategic enclave impregnable to any army with such limited resources as those possessed by the Teutonic Knights.

Six months prior to the lifting of the siege, plague struck within the walls of Allenstein Castle.

Much of the renowned astronomer's reputation at the time rested upon his skill as a physician. As a youth he had studied medicine at the University of Padua, and, although never obtaining a medical degree, he did acquire a professional proficiency reputed to be well above the level of his contempories. The specific nature of the Allenstein plague cannot now be identified, but it was a moderately serious affair with much morbidity, although only two fatalities.

Copernicus, who at first contented himself with prescribing routine treatments, became disquieted when in many instances the disease either persisted in spite of his therapy, or reappeared in cases which he regarded as cured. Rather than limit himself to ineffective treatment he decided to search out and define its aetiology and pathogenesis. News of this rather basic approach soon spread beyond Ermland and travelled as far west as Leipzig where it reached the ears of Adolph Buttenadt, who had known the young Copernicus in Padua and who had served as Copernicus' sponsor for memberhsip of the Guild of Apothecaries and Physicians.

Buttenadt, unlike Copernicus, did earn a degree in medicine but hardly ever practised. Instead he dedicated himself to informational and organisational tasks in the very powerful physicians' guild and became, in the highest sense of the word, a professional propagandist.

NICOLAS COPERNIC

Né a Thorn le 19 Février 1473. Mort a Warmie le 11 Mai 1543.

Paris chés Odieuvre m.d d'Estampes quai de l'Ecole vis à vis la Samarit. à la belle Image. C.P.

Before Copernicus the Ptolemaic concept of the universe was that all the planets orbited in perfect circles around the Earth. With Copernican theory, though, the Sun was at the centre of the universe, and not the Earth. He published this idea at the end of his life and received the first copy of his book De Revolutionibus Orbicum Coelestium *(On the Revolutions of the Heavenly Spheres) on his deathbed. Legend has it that when Copernicus read the Preface, he collapsed and died. This had been written by one of his disciples, Andreas Osiander, whom he had not bothered to mention in his own Introduction to the book. Osiander repaid this by including an unauthorised Preface explaining that what followed was pure hypothesis and need not be taken too seriously. To add insult to injury, Osiander had not even signed the Preface and so it looked as if it had been written by Copernicus himself! (Courtesy Wellcome Institute Library, London.)*

103

By 1517 he had become Grand Master of the Apothecaries of Medieval Allegmagne, which was the official name of the Northern European chapter of the Guild of Apothecaries and Physicians.

The news of Copernicus' research activities disconcerted the Grand Master and resulted in his visit to Allenstein to express his concern about events. He hoped that the reports had no basis in fact, but not only did Copernicus confess that they were true, but also revealed that he had actually discovered the cause of the Allenstein plague and had instituted measures to prevent its recurrence. Buttenadt was astonished and bewildered by this new development and contended that such activities could undermine the entire contemporary ethos of medical science. The Grand Master did not allow that in attempting good works man necessarily served as a beneficient instrument. Although he could appreciate Copernicus' noble intentions, he also suspected that these might have inadvertently altered Nature's balance and thus redirected the will of God. The latter possibility was the chief basis for his concern, which if true, he feared could occasion divine retribution. Buttenadt admitted that his fears, if put into operation, might act to suppress originality in medical science but he was only an advocate of cautious innovation.

Copernicus protested that this affair hardly justified such apprehension and to assure Buttenadt that his ministerings could have no significant impact beyond the castle, he described the activities leading to his discovery.

Suspecting some correlation between the plague and the food available at the castle, he divided the inhabitants into separate groups each with special diets. Before long it had become apparent that the small group denied bread was the only one free from plague. If it had been plausible, Copernicus would have dispensed with all use of bread, but this was difficult in a besieged castle. Christian charity had required that only those Allenstein inhabitants too old or infirm to provide for themselves be domiciled within the castle and that all able-bodied non-military residents were to withdraw from the vicinity. As a result the castle population consisted only of military personnel directly involved with defence or enfeebled peasants. The labour shortage meant that even the latter were pressed into some kind of service.

The most difficult function for this elderly and infirm group was that of occasional waiter! The military were not permitted to leave their posts during their 12-hour tours of duty and their meals during this period were brought to them by the peasants. They lacked the stamina for such work, climbing from the kitchens to the high turrets where the guards were stationed, up narrow stairways for almost 200 feet above ground level. Items of food were often dropped and though probably brushed free of the more obvious contamination were nevertheless delivered for consumption by the guards. The food most frequently dropped were the Allenstein baked bread, which were large, coarse, black loaves, which could collect substantial amounts of foreign debris without noticeable discolouration. The diet of all castle inhabitants consisted in large part of this bread.

It was then suggested to Copernicus as commander of the castle, by one Gerhard Glickselig, that the bread loaves should be coated with a thin layer of an edible light-coloured spread. After such treatment, any foreign matter adhering to fallen loaves would then be readily visible and potential plague victims would be able to protect themselves by removing the contaminated material. A decision was made to coat all bread with a spread of churned cream. This subsequently resulted in the elimination of all plague from the castle.

Buttenadt regarded the localised nature of Copernicus' clinical success as sufficiently mitigating to dispense with any necessity of discipline at his unprofessional behaviour (in the sixteenth century!). However, it was agreed that the incident should remain unpublicised.

Copernicus died in 1543, and two years after his death the Schmalkaldic War erupted and Buttenadt, who was still alive and by then executive secretary of the Guild of Apothecaries and Physicians, was appalled at the backwash of disease and pestilence which appeared in the wake of the wars throughout Europe at that time. He was desperate to prevent the rapid spread of plagues, particularly those of the Schmalkaldic War, and now broadcasted the details of the late Copernicus' Allenstein cure. As a result, the system of coating bread was rapidly adopted throughout Europe. There is no evidence that this worked in any plague other than at Allenstein but nevertheless, once adopted, the coating practice proved to be surprisingly durable and was eventually integrated into the dietary habits of the vast majority of Europeans. As an apparent tribute to its most effective proponent, it was described as *Buttenadting* which today is called *buttering*.

REFERENCES
Adapted from Hand S B and Kunin A S 1970 *J. Am. Med. Assoc.* **214** 2312–15. Additional biographical information on Copernicus from Wilson C 1980 *Starseekers* (New York: Doubleday).

Irish Proverb

The beginning of health is sleep.

Medicinal Uses of Wine

The oldest known record of the medicinal use of wine is an inscribed clay tablet excavated from the ancient Sumerian city of Nippur, south of the supposed site of Babylon. Now stored in the University of Pennsylvania Museum at Philadelphia, the tablet describes drugs made with wine. Archaeologists believe the tablet dates back to about 3000 BC.

Later, wine was a principal medicine in Greece. Homer's *Iliad* says that Machaon and Podalirius (physician sons of Asklepios, the Greek god-physician) administered wine to the wounded heroes of the Trojan War. Hippocrates of Cos (460–370 BC) also made extensive use of wine, prescribing it as a wound dressing, a cooling agent for fevers, a purgative, and a diuretic.

© American Medical Association 1977

REFERENCE
J. Am. Med. Assoc. 1977 **238** 464

Onion Incantation to Exorcise Sickness

The tablets of the Babylonians and Assyrians have preserved for posterity a long list of exorcising formulae in which various substances like onions, dates, palm clusters, bits of sheep's hide and goat skin and coloured wool are introduced to be peeled or torn to pieces, and as each bit is thrown into the fire an incantation is recited. The rite is purely symbolical and in the case of the onion is the following:

> As this onion is peeled and thrown into the fire,
> Consumed by the glowing fire-god,
> Never to be planted again in a garden,
> Never to be harrowed, never to take root,
> Will never again be placed in the ground,
> Its stalk will never grow, will never see the sunlight again,
> Will never come onto the table of a God or King,
> So may the ban curse, pain and woe,
> Sickness, groans, injury, sin, misdeed and transgression,
> So may the sickness in my body, in my flesh, in my limbs
> As this peeled onion, be consumed by the glowing fire-god.

REFERENCE
Jastrow M 1917 'Babylonian-Assyrian Medicine' *Annuals of Medical History* **1** 236

The Oyster's Consolation

(Lines suggested by an antivivisectionist's appeal against the cruelty of eating oysters alive.)

I cannot laugh, I cannot wail, I cannot even droop a tail;
I cannot say how much I feel, I cannot squirm, I cannot
  squeal.
No eye have I for mute appeal, no tears a-down a cheek to
  steal;
No brow to dew with anguished sweat, no ear to hear, no mind
  to fret.

Sprinkled with pepper black or red, I calmly lie as if in bed;
I cannot even raise a quiver when forks are bedded in my liver.
But ah! I have a dainty taste, a palate all around my waist;
So all day long to feed I strive, and swallow all my food alive.

Can I complain if hungry man adopts this very simple plan,
Meting to me the self-same measure by bolting me alive with
  pleasure?
Yet, pity me not with frantic screech, the opening knife my
  vitals reach—
Swallowed by epicure or glutton, I am stone dead, as dead as
  mutton.

REFERENCE
Rayner H 1920 *Br. Med. J.* **2** 262

Biology Exam Howlers

Edward Jenner was alive when smallpox was a popular disease.

Fertilization takes place in the Eustachian tube.

Sewage has been in existence since Roman times.

The female uterus is hidden by the pelvic gurgle.

Flies cannot live at a height of more than six feet underground.

Unwanted pregnancy is a sexually transmitted disease.

The function of the ciliary muscles is to focus rays of light onto the rectum.

TB patients should be given special care. His mistress and pillows should be put into the sun and washed with boiling water.

REFERENCE
Biologist 1982, Volume 29, p 203

Illustrations from a Twelfth-Century Medical Treatise

Latin translations are courtesy of Dorothy Mould.

Trepanning the skull, possibly for epilepsy. (Courtesy Mansell Collection.)

Diagnosis of stomach pains. In the twelfth century the anatomical position of the stomach would not necessarily be known. (Courtesy Mansell Collection.)

The language is medieval Latin and this illustration seems to refer to pain related to swellings in the armpits and possibly to breast cancer. (Courtesy Mansell Collection.)

The top part of the illustration demonstrates the method of surgical treatment of haemorrhoids, whereas the bottom part obviously refers to nosebleeds. (Courtesy Mansell Collection.)

Annointing the whites of the eyes. (Courtesy Mansell Collection.)

110

Anecdote of an Australian Professor of Physiology

Before the Second World War, all students had to pay their lecture fees to attend the university and if they failed to attend lectures, they were plainly stupid. But after the war, when the Commonwealth Reconstruction and Training Scheme was paying the fees for returned ex-servicemen and not only paying their fees, but living expenses in addition, many students took second jobs in the city and did not attend their lectures. So, the Commonwealth Reconstruction and Training Scheme offices requested the university to get the various schools at the university to call the roll to ascertain which students were not attending.

The university then got in touch with the various professors, who chaired the schools and they all agreed to call the roll. Reports then came into the university from all the various schools, with the exception of the school of physiology. After about a month, the university sent a polite note to Professor Wright, saying that he might have forgotten.

After another fortnight had gone by and still no report from the school of physiology, the university sent over a rather stronger note, saying to the Professor that he had always cooperated in the past and what was wrong now. So, on the following Monday morning, he arrived at the lecture theatre with a big roll book.

He said, 'From now on, I call the roll and any student who does not answer runs the risk of losing his CRTS allowances. He will never become a doctor, so it is absolutely essential that every student attends every lecture. Do you all understand that?

'Yes, sir.'

He then commenced to call the roll: 'Aarons K.'

'Sir.'

'Akron D.'

'Sir.'

'Arkwright J.'

'Sir.'

And he continued to call the roll, until he came to Colwell J. He said, 'Colwell J'. there was no answer. He repeated 'Colwell J' in a louder voice. Still there was no answer.

Professor Wright called out, 'Can everyone hear me in the theatre, even those right at the back?'

There was a chorus of 'Yes, Sir'.

He called out again 'Colwell J'. Still there was no answer.

Then he said, 'Hasn't the poor bugger got any friends?'

REFERENCE

Gillespie-Jones A S 1978 *The Lawyer who Laughed* (Hutchinson of Australia: Richmond, Australia) p. 44

Anecdote of a Roman Medical School, 80 AD

Asclepiades (*c*.124–40 BC) was the first Roman doctor to achieve high fame. He came to Rome from Bithynia and founded a medical school which continued after his death. At first, such schools were the personal following of the doctor and he would take all his students with him on visits. The writer Martial (40–102 AD) commented on this practice in the following manner:

> I was lying ill; but you immediately came to me, Symmacchus, accompanied by a hundred students. A hundred hands, frozen by the north wind, examined me. I did not have a fever, Symmachus, but I've got one now.

Anecdote of Nansen

During the preparations for one of his polar expeditions, Fridtjof Nansen (1861–1930) was visited by a stout man who wanted to sign on for Nansen's future expedition. The man took a seat in front of the polar investigator with his bowler bravely on top of his head. Nansen had to get good qualities in the men he hired and to test this man, he reached for a revolver, aimed at the man and pulled off a bullet through the man's hat. The latter did not react at all.

'Well, please take this money for a new hat', Nansen said.

'Thank you very much' the man answered 'but what about the trousers'.

'I have not done anything to them' said Nansen.

'Well, I have' said the man.

REFERENCE

Contributed by Arne Skretting who translated from the Norwegian the anecdote in *Alverdens Anekdoter II, 1000 Person-Anekdoter* (Politikens: Copenhagen) 1964.

Fission of Sir Arthur Conan Doyle into Sherlock Holmes and Doctor Watson

My favourite review of a TV programme is that by Nancy Banks-Smith in the *Guardian* of 11 December 1987. The TV programme was on the BBC earlier that week and was called *The Case of Sherlock Holmes*.

Conan Doyle is the visible proof that inside every fat man there is a thin one biding his time. Doyle looked a strapping tweedy chap with a moustache at the top and a dog at the bottom as you could see in the precious film clip in *The Case of Sherlock Holmes*. The very image of Dr Watson.

But what is that, round and glittering rising and falling on his substantial waistcoat? Not a fob, not a monocle. Eliminate the impossible and what remains, however improbable, must be the truth. A magnifying glass.

A hundred years ago, in a historic bit of fission, Conan Doyle split into good, old Dr Watson and Sherlock Holmes, 'Tall and slender, given to long bouts of depression relieved only by cocaine in a 7 per cent solution. A tortured as well as a lonely man.' The fall-out can still be measured.

I might mention that Dr Jekyll and Mr Hyde had been published the year before. These are deep waters, Watson.

Doyle was an Irishman whose father drank himself into an asylum, a background not dissimilar to Shaw's or Chaplin's. Geniuses are not mad but they probably know someone who is.

The case of Sherlock Holmes was a 40 Minutes Special, you could tell it was special because it lasted 70 minutes. The idea was to investigate the Holmes phenomenon and make a bit of money for the BBC. To this end it turned into a fair old international rag-bag of films and fans.

My favourite, I confess was a Czechoslovakian film in which a voluptuous woman in a sort of corset gripped the hand of Sherlock Holmes and said vibrantly, 'I hunger for you.' Her hand moved up his pale blue sleeve towards his velvet collar. 'Have you,' she added hungrily, 'your violin with you?'

'Of course.' said Holmes, 'I never go anywhere without it.'

'I love a man who gets hold of a violin by its neck,' she cried holding his hands to her pounding heart.

In America John Bennet Shaw, an undertaker who, I suspect, found his sense of humour too well developed for his job, has devoted his life to Holmes. He has the largest collection of Holmes memorabilia in the world including three chocolate rabbits called Inspector Hector ('Terrible chocolate but artistic of course') and ladies' panties with a picture of Holmes, his magnifying glass and 'It must be in here somewhere.' He is a collector, he cheerfully agrees, with the sensitivity of a vacuum cleaner.

Once a year he leads a pilgrimage to the confused hamlet of Moriarty in New Mexico. Wearing deerstalkers, they sing 'unhappy birthday to you, you bastard' (Bastard, Shaw alleges, was Moriarty's middle name) and deposit ceremonial dung. Moriarty considers it the highlight of the year but, then, there's not a helluva lot going on there the other 364 days.

At the end of a windy English pier, Paul Sparks, who has modelled his life on Holmes's methods, was wearing a helmet sprouting wire coat hangers and demonstrating a device for tracking down stolen bicycles which, one fears, is still in its infancy. Mr Sparks explained that he was 'Trying to see patterns in the chaos of life.'

When he finds one I hope he will let me know. Likewise if he finds my bicycle.

Zip Answer to Stomach Problem

People with severe internal abdominal infections run a high risk of dying if their abdominal cavities are not regularly drained. However, this is easier said than done, because draining may involve constantly opening and closing the wound.

Spanish surgeons have come up with a neat solution to this problem: they close the access with a nylon/polythene zip which can be undone every day.

A report in the *Archives of Surgery* says that doctors at the Provincial Hospital, Madrid, have been using zippers since 1982 and have successfully treated more than 60 patients either with an infected pancreas or infections following perforations of the intestine.

REFERENCE
The *Independent* 1 March 1988

Prisoner Surprises the Police Taking Him to Jail

'I have swallowed a spoon' was the amazing statement made to police who were taking Joseph Tyson, an electrician, to Preston Prison. He was removed to Preston Infirmary and examined under the x-rays, when a metallic substance was located near the stomach. An operation for its removal was performed, but Tyson still remains in the Infirmary in a serious condition. It appears that he broke off the bowl of the spoon and swallowed the shank end. He was under remand on a charge of obtaining £120 by false pretences from a woman to whom he had proposed marriage.

[X-rays were discovered in November 1895 but from the amount of press coverage of this incident it would appear that this was the first case, at least in the United Kingdom, of spoon-swallowing diagnosed by x-rays. Earlier reported swallowing incidents tended to refer to coins or false teeth.]

A set of false teeth lodged in the throat, 1902 case, 20 years before the episode with the spoon.

REFERENCE
Hull Daily News 16 March 1922

$10 000 Radium Used to Cure Sing Sing Convict

Radium worth $10 000 was taken inside the walls of Sing Sing Prison and is being used today by Dr Amos O Squire, head prison physician, to treat John Duffy, a cancer patient in the prison hospital. The radium, which is the personal property of Dr Squire, was used to try and cure Duffy, who was operated on for cancer of the lip last Saturday. Duffy was committed to Sing Sing for assault in Brooklyn. Doctors also reported that John Amishoki, the ex-convict who voluntarily returned to Sing Sing in order to continue the treatment he was receiving for a tumour of the brain, was much improved and will probably leave the prison in a few days.

REFERENCE
Brooklyn Daily Eagle 11 October 1921

The Medico-legal Significance of X-rays in the First Year after their Discovery

1 THE ACTRESS WHO FELL DOWN THE STAIRS (England)

One of the first lawsuits in which x-ray picture evidence became of great importance was heard in Nottingham in England. It was described in a number of British journals in March, 1896, and shortly thereafter was commented upon by several American journals. This case was described as follows in the *London Hospital* under the title, 'The New Photography in Court.'

> An interesting and novel case, in which the 'X-rays' practically decided the point, was tried by Mr. Justice Hawkins and a special jury at Nottingham the other day. Miss Ffolliott, a burlesque and comedy actress, while carrying out an engagement at a Nottingham theatre early in September last, was the subject of an accident. After the first act, having to go and change her dress, she fell on the staircase leading to the dressing-room and injured her foot. Miss Ffolliott remained in bed for nearly a month, and at the end of that time was still unable to resume her vocation. Then, by the advice of Dr. Frankish, she was sent to the University College Hospital, where both her feet were photographed by the 'X-rays.' The negatives taken were shown in court, and the difference between the two was convincingly demonstrated to the judge and jury. There was a definite displacement of the cuboid bone of the left foot, which showed at once both the nature and the measure of the injury. No further argument on the point was needed on either side, and the only defence, therefore, was a charge of contributory carelessness against Miss Ffolliott. Those medical men who are accustomed to dealing with 'accident claims'—and such claims are now very numerous—will perceive how great a service the new photography may render to truth and right in difficult and doubtful cases. If the whole osseous system, including the spine, can be portrayed distinctly

116

on the negative, much shameful perjury on the part of a certain class of claimants, and many discreditable contradictions among medical experts, will be avoided. The case is a distinct triumph for science, and shows how plain fact is now furnished with a novel and successful means of vindicating itself with unerring certainty against opponents of every class.

The presentation of the new 'wonder pictures' before a solemn court had varying effects. Not everyone was readily convinced of the value of such pictures for court procedures, and 'some amusing remarks were made,' said the *Journal of Photography:*

> On the defendant's counsel telling one of the witnesses that he ought to have scientific evidence as to the value of the rays, Mr. Justice Hawkins remarked, 'You might send a man to the lunatic asylum, you know, by photographing his head.' One of the barristers, looking at the photographs, asked, 'Is this the Trilby?' &c. Evidently the 'New Photography' was treated with a certain degree of levity on its first appearance as a witness, by the gentlemen of the long robe.'

2 BULLET IN THE LEG (Canada)

In April the *Medical Record* wrote under the title, 'Roentgen Rays in Court':

> The *Canadian Medical Review*, quoting from a Montreal daily paper, said that the court of Queen's Bench of that city will be the first court on record where Roentgen's new photographic discovery will be used in evidence. A photograph of the leg of Tolson Cumming, who was shot on Christmas Eve, will be filed, showing the location of the bullet. The photograph was taken by Professor Cox, of McGill University.'

3 DOCK LABOURER'S BROKEN ARM (England)

Another English case, in which x-ray plates were used as evidence, was described in July 1896, in the *British Journal of Photography* under the title, 'A County Court Judge and the Roentgen Rays.'

> At the Liverpool County Court on Monday, during the hearing of an action under the Employers' Liability Act, in which a dock labourer claimed £150 damages for personal injuries, the plaintiff's counsel produced two photographs of the injured arm taken by means of the roentgen rays. He proposed to use these photographs as evidence. The defendant's counsel objected, stating that he has no reason to believe that Dr. Buchanan, of the University College, by whom the photographs had been taken, was competent to produce reliable radiographs by the new process. Judge Shand replied that, from all he had read concerning the process, he believed that he himself should be able to take photographs by this method, providing he had the necessary apparatus. Dr. Buchanan agreed, stating that the process was perfectly

simple, and could be carried out by anyone. Judge Shand felt compelled to admit the authenticity of the photographs, but stated that the question as to their value must be discussed by the defendant's counsel and the jury. When the photographs were produced, they showed clearly the injury which had been done to the bone of plaintiff's arm and the jury awarded the plaintiff £60 damages.

In June a detailed discussion of the legal significance of Roentgen pictures appeared in the *British Medical Journal.*

4 WIFE MURDER (England)

The radiograph is thought to be of one of the bullets fired by Hargreaves Hartley into the brain of his wife Elizabeth Ann Hartley at Nelson, Lancashire, on 23 April 1896, and 'photographed with x-rays' by the then Professor of Physics at Manchester University, Sir Arthur Schuster, on 2 May 1896.

5 TROLLEY CAR ACCIDENT (USA)

W J Morton, in his book *The X-ray*, stated in September 1896:

> A very important application of the x-ray will be in connection with expert testimony in the court. Court records contain numerous cases in which the x-ray would have been of great service. Already it has been used for this purpose. I have a picture of the knees of a person which is likely to find its way into court. The patient was thrown down with violence in a trolley-car accident more than a year ago, and has suffered more or less ever since. An exposure was first made of the injured knee only and afforded no positive evidence of the seat or degree of the injury. By resorting to the comparative method, a picture of both knees was obtained which showed that the upper portion of the large bone of the leg below the knee was nearly three-quarters of an inch wider in the injured knee than in the normal one. This was doubtless due to fracture and subsequent growth of bone. Such a picture is very convincing and would be sure to have great weight with a jury.

Note: The original x-ray negative is now a court record and it is impossible to obtain possession of the same to make a half-tone reproduction until the case is settled. The picture will be reproduced in future editions of this work as soon as the original negative can be obtained.

6 SURGEON LOSES MALPRACTICE CASE (France)

At about the same time [as case 5 above] the *Journal of the American Medical Association* reported the use of x-ray plates in a trial in France as follows:

> We note that at the trial of an action for damages at Nancy, in France, the surgeon who had charge of the injured plaintiff was accused of having caused the damage by mistaking a dislocation for a fracture. The accusation was sustained by producing in court a roentgen photograph which showed clearly the bones in the dislocated position without a fracture.

The physician lost the suit.

7 ATTEMPTED MURDER (England)

An interesting use of x-rays in a case of attempted murder was also described in the English *Journal of Photography*.

> Henry Goodwin was again brought up last week at the Salford Police Court, and charged before Mr R Hankinson and Mr Alderman Jenkins with burglary and attempting to murder Mr Israel Rosenblum,

merchant, Northumberland Street, Higher Broughton. Prisoner was remanded for another week on the application of Chief Detective Inspector Lyogue, who said that there was now a likelihood of Mr Rosemblum's recovery, but he would not be in a fit state to attend court for two or three weeks. In the course of an interview, Dr Walmsley, the medical attendant of Mr Rosenblum, stated that his patient had been photographed by roentgen rays by Mr Chadwick, of St Mary's Street, and, as the result of the process, the bullet was discovered in the chest. An operation with a view to its extraction will be made in the course of a few days.

8 TERRORIST BOMBS (France)

The etching shows Post Office or Customs staff in the surroundings of a railway station examining a package. This use of x-rays had been described by Snowden Ward in 1896 to 'reveal the contents of certain suspected packets, which have proved to be infernal machines'. It is not known if this led to cases in the law courts.

9 THE LAW STUDENT WHO FELL OFF A LADDER (USA)

Towards the end of the year a law suit came up in Denver, Colorado, in which, again, roentgen-ray pictures were admitted as evidence. 'The suit was brought April 14, 1896, by one, James Smith, a poor boy who was reading law and doing odd jobs to see his expenses. He was injured in a fall from a ladder and after some time he consulted

120

a well-known surgeon, who made no attempt at immobilization of the thigh, but advised exercise of various kinds as though treating a contusion.' The trial came up on December 2, 1896; the Judge was Owen E LeFevre, the Prosecutors for J Smith, Plaintiff, were B B Lindsey and N F W Parks. They qualified one H H Buckwalter as an expert in photography and in the use of roentgen rays because he had been making x-ray shadow-graphs for the past eight months. Plates of J Smith were made November 7, 11, 21 and 28, 1896. The most satisfactory one required an exposure of eighty minutes.

Judge Lindsey said that he had been in personal communication with Judges in the East who had refused to accept x-ray plates in evidence, and that one of them had stated to him that he had sustained an objection to the offering of x-ray plates in evidence, 'because,' said he, 'there is no proof that such a thing is possible. It is like offering the photograph of a ghost,' continued the judge 'when there is no proof that there is any such thing as a ghost.' In order to convey the idea of radiographic shadows to the Judge and the jury, Buckwalter, Lindsey and Parks contrived a shadow box and showed an ordinary shadow picture and then an x-ray shadowgraph of a hand. Next the shadow of a normal femur was shown and then the roentgen shadowgraph of such a femur and finally there was shown the x-ray plate of a picture of the plaintiff's left femur. This radiograph showed that the head of the bone was not in normal relationship to the great trochanter and the shaft, and it was proposed by the prosecutor that this radiograph be submitted to the jury as evidence that there had been a fracture of the femur in the region of the great trochanter with impaction of the fragments. C J Hughes, a Denver lawyer, argued for the defence for more than three hours against the admission of such evidence, stating that 'X-ray photographs' are not admissable under the law and past decisions of the court bore this out. He contended, furthermore, that even should it be admitted this was a photograph of J Smith's femur, so it could not be used as competent testimony under the broad principle of the law upon the matter of photographs as testimony because witnesses must testify to having seen the object which had been photographed and to having identified the photograph as a good likeness of the object—then only may any photograph be admitted as evidence.

On the following morning Judge LeFevre expressed his opinion on the exhibits consisting of 4 × 6 plates. (*Denver Republican*, Thursday, December 2, 1896.)

'The defendant's counsel objected to the admission in evidence of exhibits, the same being photographs produced by means of X-ray process, on the ground that, being photographs of an object unseen by the human eye, there is no evidence that the photograph accurately portrays and represents the object so photographed. This rule of law is well settled by a long line of authorities and we do not dissent therefrom as applied to photographs which may be seen by the human eye. The reason of this salutary rule is so apparent to the profession that as a rule of evidence we will not discuss it.

We, however, have been presented with a photograph taken by means of a new scientific discovery, the same being acknowledged in the arts and in science. It knocks for admission at the temple of learning; what shall we do or say? Close fast the doors or open wide the portals?

These photographs are offered in evidence to show the present condition of the head and neck of the femur bone which is entirely hidden from the eye of the surgeon. Nature has surrounded it with tissues for its protection and there it is hidden; it cannot by any possibility be removed nor exposed that it may be compared with its shadow as developed by means of this new scientific process.

In addition to these exhibits in evidence, we have nothing to do or say as to what they purport to represent; that will, without doubt, be explained by eminent surgeons. These exhibits are only pictures or maps to be used in explanation of a present condition, and therefore are secondary evidence, and not primary. They may be shown to the jury as illustrating or making clear the testimony of experts.

The law is the acme of learning throughout all ages. It is the essence of wisdom, reason and experience. Learned priests have interpreted the law, have classified reasons for certain opinions which, in time, have become precedents, and these ordinarily guide and control especially trial courts. We must not, however, hedge ourselves round about with rule, precept and precedent until we can advance no farther; our field must ever grow, as trade, the arts and science seek to enter it.

During the last decade, at least, no science has made such mighty strides forward as surgery. It is eminently a scientific profession, alike interesting to the learned and unlearned. It makes use of all science and learning. It has been of inestimable service to mankind. It must not be said of the law that it is wedded to precedent; that it will not lend a helping hand. Rather, let the courts throw open the door to all well-considered scientific discoveries. Modern science has made it possible to look beneath the tissues of the human body, and has aided surgery in telling of the hidden mysteries. We believe it to be our duty in this case to be the first, if you please to so consider it, in admitting in evidence a process known and acknowledged as a determinate science. The exhibits will be admitted in evidence.

In telling of the trial, Judge Lindsey stated: 'The electrical apparatus, batteries, Crookes tube, etc., were all in the court-room. We offered to show the jury the bones in their hands, which created such terrific excitement about the court-house that extra bailiffs were called in to keep the court in order during the argument. The excitement was intense, the 'gallery' on my side restrained from breaking into applause on several occasions because of their anxiety to have this 'miracle' demonstrated and actually recognized by a court.'

10 X-RAYS AND DIVORCE CASES (England)

The alacrity with which the medical and the judicial professions took up the new discovery of Röntgen and made use of it as evidence in court trials is remarkable. It is not surprising then that some persons less concerned with truth looked upon the use of the x-ray for more or less fraudulent purposes. On August 8, 1896, the London *Standard* carried the following advertisment: 'The New Photography—Owing to the success Mr Henry Slater has personally achieved with the New Photography, he is prepared to introduce same in divorce matters free of charge. Offices, No. 1, Basinghall Street, City.'

How the roentgen rays could be used for the purposes of clearing up divorce matters was not exactly explained, but a theory was propounded by the editor of the *Electrical Engineer*, who wrote on September 8, 1896:

> Mr. Slater, as a detective, is evidently up to date. We presume he uses the X-ray to discover the skeleton which every closet is said to contain. Ability to do the detective act without squinting through a keyhole is regarded evidently as one of the recommendations of the rays, which themselves prefer darkness rather than light.

REFERENCES
Case histories 1–3, 5–7, 9–10: Glasser O 1933 *Wilhelm Conrad Röntgen and the Early History of Roentgen Rays* (John Bale, Sons & Danielsson Ltd: London)
Case histories 4, 8: Mould R F 1980 *A History of X-rays and Radium* (IPC Business Press: Sutton)

The Duc de Richelieu on Handwriting

If you gave me six sentences written by the most innocent of men, I will find something in them with which to hang him.

Lord Palmerston's Last Words

Die, my dear doctor. That's the last thing I shall do.

Radiation Protection in 1910

REFERENCE
X-ray equipment catalogue of Newton & Company, London

A Specialist

Choose your specialist and you choose your disease.

REFERENCE
The Westminster Review 18 May 1906

124

Persian Anatomy

Persian anatomical drawing showing the arterial system. (Courtesy Wellcome Institute Library, London.)

Philosophy

Philosophy like medicine, has plenty of drugs, few good remedies and hardly any specific cures.
Nicholas Chamfort (1741–1794)

Varicose Veins in Ancient Greece

Votive relief of a man holding a huge leg showing varicose veins. From the Asklepion, Athens and now in the National Museum, Athens. (Courtesy Wellcome Institute Library, London.)

An Adult

An adult is one who has ceased to grow vertically but not horizontally.

George Washington's Medical Supplies

In the bicentennial issue of the *Journal of the American Medical Association* many fascinating historical articles were published including one about an American physician in 1776. Within this text it was stated:

> The following order for medical supplies for his family and slaves at Mount Vernon was placed by George Washington with his London factor in 1767
>
> 2 best Lancets in one case
> 6 Common Do. [lancets] each in sepe. [separate case?]
> 25 lb. Antimony [used as an emetic]
> 10 lb. flour of Sulphur [an aperient]
> 2 Oz. Honey Water. [pectoral]
> 3 Quarts Spirits of Turpentine. [stimulant]
> 2 lb. best Jesuit's Bark, powdered. [quinine, used as a tonic and antiseptic]
> 3 Oz. Rhubarb Do. [powdered] and put into a bottle. [cathartic]
> 1 pint Spirit of Hartshorn [ammonia, a stimulant]
> 6 Do. Do. Nitre [diuretic and febrifuge]
> 1 lb. Blistering Plaister [made from Cantharides]
> 4 Oz. Tincture of Castor. [purgative]
> 8 Do. Balsam Capivi [copaiba, a corroborant, stimulant and diaphoretic]
> 1–4 lb. Termerick [Turmeric, a condiment used in curry; substitute for saffron]

© American Medical Association 1976

REFERENCE
Journal of the American Medical Association 1976 **236** 28

Derbes's Law

(Contributed by Dr Vincent J Derbes of New Orleans.)

Most of our pleasures come from filling or emptying cavities, and vice versa.

THE BUCK-PASSING MACHINE

FENCE FOR SITTING ON

CAT
(For not letting out of the bag)

CAN CARR
DEVICE

PULL & FLUSH Ltd

to be filled by audit sec.

AUDIT SECTION PROJECT SHOOTING GUN

BRANDY & OXYGEN CYLINDERS
(For those forced to make a decision)

RESIGNATOR PLUNGER
(Or "I'm leaving at the end of the week" indicator)

LAST RESORT SHELF
(Contents include books on "opportunities in the National Health Service" & a timetable for the Trans-Siberian Express)

THE SCREW JACK
(For use with Government Statistics)

THE HYDRAULIC JACK
(For bringing one down to earth gently)

IN TRAY

OUT

500 METRE R OF GOVERNM MEMORAND SHEETS

THE I'M ALL RIGHT JACK

HIGH FREQUENCY CHECKING VALVE
(For checking the checker who checks the checker's checker)

CLANGER DROPPING GEAR

FLAP SUPPRESSOR LEVER

PASSED TO YOU

PASSED TO THEM

PASSED TO HIM

Special fading ink

HELIOGRATIATOR & GANAGULATOR SWITCH
(Automatically blames it on the bloke who left last year)

GROGGLE BOX CONTROL
(Or simple-issue complicator system)

ASHCAN FOR SALARY RISE REQUESTS FROM PHYSICISTS & ENGINEERS

DEVICE FOR WRITING ILLEGIBLE SIGNATURES

SPECIAL WIPER
(For keeping desk clear)

SMELLING SALTS
(For use when asked to sign something)

Seeking Health in Babylon

'Seeking Health'. Suppliants approaching a shrine, the door of which stands open. Sketch of an impression from an early dynastic Assyro-Babylonian cylinder seal, c. *2800* BC. *(Courtesy Wellcome Institute Library, London.)*

The Pigtail of Li-Fang-Fu

The two British Music Hall comic monologues about doctors and hospitals which were included in *Mould's Medical Anecdotes* were well received and consequently a further two have been placed in this volume. This time the monologues concern that favourite topic of comedians—Death. Many are set in exotic places such as India and the Far East, such as this example of 'The Pigtail of Li-Fang-Fu' which involves opium addiction. The second example (p. 155) is just called 'Suicide', but it is far from morbid! 'The Pigtail' was written by Sax Rohmer and T W Thurban in 1919.

> They speak of a dead man's vengeance; they whisper a
>   deed of hell
>   'Neath the Mosque of Mohammed Ali.
>   And this is the thing they tell.
> In a deep and a midnight gully, by the street where the
>   goldsmiths are,
>   'Neath the Mosque of Mohammed Ali, at the back of
>   the Scent Bazaar,

Was the House of a Hundred Raptures, the tomb of a
    thousand sighs;
    Where the sleepers lay in that living death which the
    opium-smoker dies.
At the House of a Hundred Raptures, where the reek
    of the joss-stick rose
    From the knees of the golden idol to the tip of his
    gilded nose,
Through the billowing oily vapour, the smoke of the
    black *chandu*,
    There a lantern green cast a serpent sheen on the
    pigtail of Li-Fang-Fu.
There was Ramsa Lal of Bhiwâni, who could smoke
    more than any three,
    A pair of Kashmiri dancing girls and Ameer Khân
    Môtee;
And there was a grey-haired soldier too, the wreck of a
    splendid man;
    When the place was still I've heard mounted drill
    being muttered by 'Captain Dan'.
Then, one night as I lay a-dreaming, there was
    shuddering, frenzied screams;
    But the smoke had a spell upon me; I was chained to
    that couch of dreams.
All my strength, all my will had left me, because of the
    black *chandu*,
    And upon the floor, by the close-barred door, lay the
    daughter of Li-Fang-Fu.
'Twas the first time I ever saw her, but often I dream
    of her now;
    For she was as sweet as a lotus, with the grace of a
    willow bough.
The daintiest ivory maiden that ever a man called fair,
    And I saw blood drip where Li-Fang-Fu's whip had
    tattered her shoulders bare!
I fought for the power to curse him—and never a
    word would come!
    To reach him—to kill him—but opium had
    stricken me helpless—dumb.
He lashed her again and again, until she uttered a
    moaning prayer,
    And as he whipped so the red blood dripped from
    those ivory shoulders bare.
When crash! went the window behind me, and in leapt
    a greyhaired man,
    As he tore the whip from that devil's grip, I knew
    him: 'twas Captain Dan!
Ne'er a word spoke he, but remorseless, grim, his brow

131

with anger black.

He lashed and lashed till the shirt was slashed from
the Chinaman's writhing back.

And when in his grasp the whip broke short, he cut
with a long keen knife.

The pigtail, for which a Chinaman would barter his
gold, his life—

He cut the pig-tail from Li-Fang-Fu. And this is the
thing they tell

By the Mosque of Mohammed Ali—for it led to a
deed of hell.

In his terrible icy passsion, Captain Dan that pig-tail
plied,

And with it he thrashed the Chinaman, until any but
he had died—

Until Li-Fang-Fu dropped limply down too feeble, it
seemed, to stand.

But swift to arise, with death in his eyes—and the
long keen knife in his hand!

Like fiends of an opium vision they closed in a fight
for life,

And nearer the breast of the Captain crept the blade
of the gleaming knife.

Then a shot! a groan—and a wisp of smoke. I
swooned and knew no more—

Save that Li-Fang-Fu lay silent and still in a red pool
near the door.

But never shall I remember how that curtain of sleep
was drawn

And I woke, 'mid a deathly silence, in the darkness
before the dawn.

There was blood on the golden idol! My God! that
dream was true!

For there, like a slumbering serpent, lay the pigtail
of Li-Fang-Fu.

From the House of a Hundred Raptures I crept ere the
news should spread

That the Devil's due had claimed Li-Fang-Fu, and
that Li-Fang-Fu was dead.

'Twas the end of that Indian summer, when Fate—or
the ancient ties—

Drew my steps again to the gully, to the Tomb of a
Thousand Sighs;

And the door of the house was open! All the blood in
my heart grew cold.

For within sat the golden idol, and he leered as he
leered of old!

And I thought that his eyes were moving in a sinister
    vile grimace
    When suddenly, there at his feet I saw a staring and
        well-known face!
With the shriek of a soul in torment, I turned like a
    frenzied man,
    Falling back from the spot where the moonlight
        poured down upon 'Captain Dan'!
He was dead, and in death was fearful; with features of
    ghastly hue—
    And snakelike around his throat was wound the
        pigtail of Li-Fang-Fu!

REFERENCE

Marshall M (ed) 1981 *The Book of Comic and Dramatic Monologues* (London: Elm Tree Books/EMI Publishing). Reproduced by permission of EMI Music Publishing Ltd.

Camel Ambulance in Afghanistan

AFGHANISTAN—A CAMEL AMBULANCE AT KURRUM

This engraving is circa 1880 and shows a camel ambulance at Kurrum during the Afghan War. (Courtesy Mary Evans Picture Library.)

Koko for the Hair

(Courtesy Mary Evans Picture Library.)

This advertisment appeared in the *Penny Pictorial Magazine*, *c.* 1900, and included a special offer for those who have not yet tried Koko—a 4/6 Trial Bottle for 2/–. The makers, The Koko-Maricopas Co of Bevis Marks, London, stated that 'We find it better to thus practically give away one bottle to make a customer than to spend large amounts on advertising'. However, they did issue another advertisement with complimentary remarks from: one John Strange Winter, the now long-forgotten author of 'Bootle's Baby', who claims it stopped his hair falling out (maybe due to worry of finding publishers for his stories!); from someone purporting to act for HRH Princess Victoria begging to send six bottle of Koko for this grandaughter of Queen Victoria; from HRH Princess Marie of Greece at the Palais Royal, Athens, to say she is very pleased with her hair; and finally, the most intriguing testimonial, from a Rear-Admiral A. Tinklar, at the address of Governor's House, H.M. Prison, Birmingham, who was very pleased with his bottle of Koko, claiming it to be a most excellent preparation. It is not stated whether this was first-hand knowledge, or whether it was somehow tested on the prisoners in Birmingham Jail!

It's not What you Write—It's the Way that you Write it

It was a lazy July morning—bang in the middle of what people in the media call the 'silly' season.

Sifting through his morning mail, the Editor of the newspaper I worked for picked up three confidential letters unopened by his secretary and, knowing my penchant for analysing people's handwriting, gave them to me.

'Here' he said. 'I haven't the vaguest idea who these are from, and I don't want to open them for a minute or two; so what can you tell me about them first?'

I examined the three envelopes briefly. Then I put my head on the chopping block.

The first was an intelligent hand; educated; from someone of high morals and principles. The writer was articulate, generous and just a shade aloof. Health was definitely not top line. I detected signs of a chronic heart condition. It was difficult to say much more from the few words on the envelope.

The second sample disturbed me. It was blatantly obvious that here was a very disturbed person. The writing crawled all over the place. The more I studied it, the more uneasy I became.

Schizoid tendencies were apparent and, I hesitated to say so, but felt

135

instinctively that here was a potential suicide who needed professional surveillance.

Number three was neat and small. A tidy hand, from a tidy mind. Definitely from someone with keen powers of concentration, analytical, with good organisational ability.

But why so utterly frustrated in every way . . . even in relation to sex?

I handed back to my Editor his three unopened envelopes and, as he ripped them apart and read the contents, I watched his expression change from one of amazement to sheer incredulity.

He placed the first on his desk, gasping 'Good God!'—which was rather apt in view of the fact that it was from the Bishop.

'You're right about his being intelligent, educated and a man of high morals and principles. Aloof? Yes, I suppose he is that, too. A heart condition, you say? It's the first I've heard. To the best of my knowledge, he's perfectly healthy.'

One down, two to go.

As he read the contents of the second, he blanched. It was a patient in the local psychiatric hospital: a hopeless schizophrenic. He was writing to say that since he had recently developed a ray of gold light around his body, he could only assume that he was 'the long-awaited Messiah.'

And so to number three, for a little light relief:

My wicked Editor was rather tickled to announce that it was from a nun; a maths mistress at a grammar school in the next county.

About to renounce her vows, she was seeking some advice about accommodation and employment. She wondered if there were any openings for trainee journalists on our paper . . . while I wondered if there any chance of having my salary doubled.

The answer in each case was, unfortunately, no.

A month passed and, in the hustle and bustle of writing copy, I forgot about the saga of the three letters. Then, out of the blue, a newsflash came in. The Bishop had had a coronary.

A week or so later, the analysis of the hospital patient was also confirmed. Deeply upset because none of those in his immediate environment afforded him the deification he felt was his right, he hanged himself from a tree in the hospital grounds.

Can the future be foretold by graphology then?

No, although it may look like it from this little sequence of events, that conclusion must be entirely ruled out. The answer is much more simple than prophecy, precognition, clairvoyance or anything else you wish to call it.

Dominant factors in the Bishop's writing showed that all was not well in the region of his heart. The break in his script at the same point was repeated again and again.

It was obviously not a slip of the pen, because there were no breaks anywhere else.

The irregularity of his heart beat produced that unmistakeable 'jump' in the writing which most graphologists would recognise for what it was.

And the mentally disturbed man?

The downward slope of his writing was a clear indication of depression. Almost every symbol in that writing spelt despair. There wasn't a glimmer of hope to be seen anywhere.

Handwriting is not merely a case of the hand moving the pen. It is directly related to the motor mechanisms of the brain.

Suppose, for the sake of argument, you were unfortunate enough to lose the use of your right arm (or the left, if that's the hand you write with) and had to make its opposite partner take over.

You would find that, once you'd got the hang of it, your style of writing would not have changed very much.

So, having established that the way you write is connected with the way your unconscious nervous system functions: one can safely assume that a slip of the pen can be as revealing as a slip of the tongue.

General mentality, long-standing illness, physical and mental handicap show up easily. Sex doesn't, though sexuality—or the lack of it—usually does.

Depressives give themselves away easily. The way in which that psychiatric patient scored through his name was almost an unconscious desire to score through himself—which, predictably, he did.

Age is difficult as a rule, unless the writing is that of a young child, or of someone very old.

So what do we look for in someone's handwriting, in order to see how they function as individuals?

Various signs and symbols—the slope of the writing, its pressure, how large (or small) are the capitals in relation to the rest of the text, and whether they are entangled with the letters above, or below.

What is the spacing like between letters, words, lines?

Are the t-strokes and i-dots all in the right place? Are they there at all?

Corroborative evidence is essential.

Pencils and felt tips can be messy. Ballpoints are better, but there is nothing like a good fountain pen to produce a clean, legible script.

Small writing shows keen powers of concentration; the large variety can be from someone who is broadminded, self-assured. Equally, a small hand could come from an obsessively tidy housewife; a large one from a flamboyant megalomaniac.

One must never jump to conclusions. There are so many factors to take into account. Does the signature differ in style from the rest of the text? Is the surname the same size as the Christian name? Are some of its letters larger than others? Does it trail off to a line, or become enlarged and have a full stop after it?

Self-importance, pride in one's spouse, strange eccentricities, diplomacy could all be evident here.

Where did the art (or science) of graphology begin? It is generally believed that Dr Camillo Baldi, Professor of Theoretical Medicine at the University of Bologna in the eighteenth century, was the man who set the wheels—or was it the quills?—in motion.

During the next 100 years or so, the concept of drawing connections between personality and handwriting was taken up by a variety of scientists throughout Europe.

Towards the end of the nineteenth century, graphology was shown to have a possible relationship with psychology and physiology.

Beavering away in Germany, Doctors William Preyer and Hans Busse produced many fascinating periodicals on the subject and were helped by two more medical men—George Meyer and Ludwig Klages; who showed that it was possible, through handwriting, to pick out indications of ill-health.

Klages became the Freud of handwriting analysis and today is either regarded as the best thing since ballpoints, or his theories are thrown out with the (inky?) bathwater.

Today, mainly in America and Scandinavia, research is being conducted into how certain illnesses manifest themselves in one's writing. While in Britain, medical scientists are also beginning to accept graphology as an aid to conventional diagnosis.

On a personal level, I use any talent I might have, to assist my husband, a busy hypnotherapist. I can tell at a glance which of his letters are from patients in real need of help. Between us, we can establish a priority list and slot in the urgent cases quickly.

And the strange thing is that patients, once they have been successfully treated, change their handwriting accordingly. Nervous, spikey scripts become more rounded as repressions are cleared and emotions brought to the fore. The backward slant of the shy introvert straightens and leans forward as the writer becomes more confident and begins to mix socially. A whole host of other changes take place until the hand is that of a healthy, well-adjusted individual.

Though maybe that's not so strange, when you consider that the purpose of hypnotherapy is to put you in tune with your own subconscious, to iron out frustrations and phobias.

Ah yes, the nun.

I hadn't forgotten, but forgive me if I don't publicise details of how

138

I detected her problem. Otherwise, you'll all be examining each other's writing and having little private chuckles if you find those tell-tale signs.

REFERENCE
Harding M 1982 *Choice Magazine* (May) pp 36–7

Is Graphology Accurate? Ask Lord Nelson and the Duke of Wellington

by Harold Winter, Monica Harding and R F Mould

INTRODUCTION

When I was interviewed about *Mould's Medical Anecdotes* for the *Liverpool Echo*, the journalist, Monica Harding, turned out to also be a graphologist (see the previous anecdote) and unexpectedly gave me a reading when I inscribed my book! However, I was able to turn the tables by obtaining her agreement to a *blind trial* of her graphology prowess using some handwriting samples that one of us (HW) had recently obtained when cataloguing some hundreds of documents in an unpublished collection containing papers relating to the political life of the early nineteenth century and to the East India Company.

The conditions of the trial were:

(1) Glossy photographs of samples of handwriting, such as a few lines of a letter or an addressed envelope, to be provided with the signature and the address of the writer deleted.

(2) Any words in the handwriting sample which might provide a clue to the writer shall be deleted.

(3) The graphology reading for each sample shall include, when possible, a description of the attributes and health of the writer together with any general comments.

(4) It is agreed that the age and sex of the writer cannot be determined from graphology.

(5) The material for the study shall be posted and returned by recorded delivery, arriving in Liverpool on 3 August and being returned to London by 6 August 1984.

All conditions were fulfilled, and in addition Monica Harding was not told that the samples were from the early nineteenth century.

LORD NELSON, 1758–1805

Engraving of Lord Nelson from a portrait by J Hoppner. (Courtesy Mansell Collection.)

It was by chance that I saw the signature on the envelope and realised that this almost illegible signature *Nelson & Bronte* was in fact that of Lord Nelson, who was also created Duke of Bronte in Sicily. The address *Merton* is Nelson's country home, Merton Place, near London, which had been bought by Emma, Lady Hamilton on Nelson's instruction. The Dr Fisher of Christ's College was a Fellow of the College at that time and he appears to have been a lawyer who died in

140

1814 at the age of 65. The reason for Nelson's communication is not known, but Fisher was quite prominent in College affairs and the Nelson family had a long connection with Christ's. Nelson's brother, the second Lord Nelson, Nelson's younger brother Suckling and his son Horatio were all members of the College.

An example (actual size) of the handwriting of Admiral Lord Nelson. If compared with the style of writing in his last letter to Lady Hamilton, written off Cadiz in October 1805 before the Battle of Trafalgar, it is at once obvious by comparing individual letters that the above sample is an original. His last letter to Lady Hamilton is in the British Museum and has been reproduced in Hattersley's biography[1] of Nelson.

From engravings in the Mansell Collection it is seen that Nelson's signature was variously Nelson, Horatio Nelson or Nelson & Bronte. These signatures with his left hand, though, are more common than those with his right hand before it was shot off by the Spaniards at Tenerife in 1797. Indeed, at a recent sale of signatures at an autograph hunter's fair in London,[2] Horatio Nelson in right-hand signature was sold for £1250. This compared with £200 for a signed photograph of Winston Churchill and £180 for a cheque signed by Charles Dickens.

For the graphology trial the word Merton, the date 1805 and the signature were omitted from the handwriting sample.

The symbol Z on the envelope is thought to indicate that the writer had not paid the postage and that the recipient, Dr Fisher, was expected to pay. This was before the days of postage stamps, the penny black and penny red, and if the letter was prepaid then a symbol was printed on the envelope which consisted of a circle surmounted by a crown and three lines of writing, for example

FREE
3 AP 3
1832

The colour of the printing was red/brown.

GRAPHOLOGY READING for Lord Nelson

The writer is proud and fiercely independent, to his own detriment. Moody—one has the impression, metaphorically speaking, that he is 'banging his head against a brick wall'. A divergent thinker who tends to live in 'cloud cuckoo land'. Totally apart from others. For this man, time is precious and not to be wasted on non-essentials. He considers there is important work to be done and believes he is the one to do it. Nor will he let go until he has completed his task: that for which he believes he was put on this earth. All of which makes life rather difficult for those around him. Bureaucracy be blowed, the 'people who matter' must take up where he leaves off. Note the determination expressed in his prolonged strokes. These are extended just enough to make their presence felt, but not so far as to become superfluous, so as to impress the masses. The final e, for example, ended rather more sharply than the writer intended, so he has added an extension, to ensure that those who read his words are quite clear about their meaning. Likewise, the capital C reinforces his innate desire to be understood by the intelligentsia.

It is my considered opinion that Alexander Pope must have known someone like this when he penned those immortal lines in his Essay on Criticism: 'Great wits are sure to madness near allied, and thin partitions do their bounds divide'. Here indeed is a *great wit*.

On health: 'Muddy' look could indicate changes in the writer's emotional state. However, I would need to see considerably more of it to determine whether this is due to epilepsy, alcoholism or some other serious cause of mental disturbance. It is also possible that the writer could be somewhat myopic. The grotesque formation of the second capital D certainly suggests some impairment. [The graphologist did not realise that the second D was the shorthand notation for Christ's.] Other interpretations of that thick, heavy stroke—a sensous nature; a strong, energetic drive in youth. Sexual activities appear normal, if spasmodic.

COMMENTARY ON THE READING

The graphology reading for Nelson is remarkable. 'Bureaucracy be blowed' recalls the incident of the telescope to the blind eye, and the

Nelsonian remark 'I see no ships'. That Nelson was proud, independent and difficult to work with is not open to doubt. The comment about the one-eyed admiral being myopic is very good at first glance, although it seems that this was prompted by a misreading of nineteenth-century shorthand notation.

A graphology reading is relevant to the date at which the handwriting sample was written. In Nelson's case this was 5 September 1805, which according to the *Encyclopaedia Britannica* must only have been a mere 10 days before he sailed from Spithead for the Battle of Trafalgar:

> When his orders came, Nelson made his emotional farewell to Emma and Horatia, his daughter by her, and on September 15 sailed from Spithead in the Victory.[3]

What price the graphologist's comment about a muddy look to the writing that could indicate changes in the writer's emotional state? Finally, her comment that Nelson's sex life was normal, if spasmodic. As an eighteenth-century sailor, it would have had to be spasmodic, at least with Lady Hamilton!

THE DUKE OF WELLINGTON, 1769–1852

Arthur Wellesley, fourth son of the first Earl of Mornington, an Irish peer, was created Earl of Wellington in 1812, the year of the battle of Badajoz at which this sketch was drawn. Later that year, after the victory of Salamanca and entry into Madrid, he was elevated to Marquis. His most famous success was, of course, Waterloo in 1815, after which he took to politics. He was Prime Minister from 1828–30, when he resigned office rather than accept parliamentary reform. He was Lord Warden of the Cinque Ports from 1829–52 and the letter used in this graphology trial, written from Walmer Castle, was therefore penned at the very start of his Wardenship.

The complete Wellington letter is shown (actual size), but for the trial, the text supplied was only:

presents his Compliments

and begs to acknowledge
the receipt of this memorial
to which
return an Answer after
reference to some Papers in
London—

On the folded piece of writing paper which formed the envelope there was written the words *From the Duke of Wellington 1829*. The handwriting in this letter is consistent with that of Wellington's letter of 9 August 1815, written in Paris to Lord Beresford less than two months after Waterloo, in which he states: 'The Battle of Waterloo was certainly the hardest fought that has been for many years I believe, and has placed in the power of the Allies the most important results'. He continues with a statement that the advantages which could stem from these results are now being wasted. This is not the only time in history that claims are made that the fruits of war are being squandered in the subsequent peace, but it also shows Wellington as other than a bloodthirsty soldier and several of his biographies emphasise the humane side to the man. There is, for example, the Duke's often quoted remark after the battle when he was given the long list of casualties:

Well, thank God I don't know what it is to lose a battle; but certainly nothing can be more painful than to gain one with the loss of so many of one's friends.

GRAPHOLOGY READING FOR THE DUKE OF WELLINGTON

The pronounced rightward slant shows someone with a lively, outgoing personality. Tightened upper loops suggest inhibition, allied

Walmer Castle Aug 28th 18—

The Duke of Wellington presents His Compliments to Sir John Scott Lillie and begs leave to acknowledge the receipt of His Memorial to which the Duke will return an Answer after reference to some Papers in London —

to bowed t strokes, one senses an ability on the part of the writer to keep his basic urges under control. Naked rompings and orgies taking place all around him would leave him unmoved. Mental exhaustion shows itself in those line droppings, *acknowledge* in line 2 and *memorial* in line 3. Lower zones don't figure very prominently, indicating that appetites are small, both sexual and food. He eats to live rather than lives to eat, which is all very honourable and worthy. Considering the d in line 2, the capital letter M in line 3 and the capital letter A in line 5, all have an historic feel. This, like the other samples in the trial, is probably the hand of someone long dead. Upper zones are dominant throughout showing the writer to have been cerebral. Looped capital L in *London* hints at some personal vanity but not enough to have the writer awfully concerned about his personal image. In the words compliments, line 1, papers, line 6 and London, line 7, the upper loop of the lower case letters rises higher than the top of the capitals which in my experience inevitably means subjugation by siblings/parents in childhood. That is, the writer's confidence and abilities were undermined as a child, resulting in an extra special effort to make a success of life later. This is simply to prove those siblings/parents wrong, or maybe simply to gain their respect.

Yes, there is real repression here, of the 21 letter e's in the sample, all except two are blackened. These are memorial in line 3 and reference in line 6.

The writer has a habit of tying himself up in knots (see the following words, at, line 3, answer, line 5, to, lines 4 and 6) but gains a certain amount of pleasure in extricating himseslf from the same knots. It is almost as if it were deliberate, to illustrate his own cleverness to lesser mortals, or to those who once undermined him.

The occasional backward loops or letters already mentioned, and, in line 2, at, in line 3, suggest mother-influence or even mother-dominance. (I've seen a similar phenomenon in the youthful hand of Prince Charles.) All of this makes me wonder if this writer was very heavily influenced by his mother. The very high capital letter M in line 3 seems to suggest it. The little tick before he goes into the letter proper is also revealing and is seen in only two places, capitals M and A. Mother-influence is strong indeed if he has to take an unconscious breather before he even pens the letter. What *did* she do to him when he was young? Now let us turn to letter A. Was there some ghastly maiden aunt also wielding her influence over him? Let us just say the lady had such an effect on him that he subsequently found it very difficult to express, indeed, feel, emotions. If he ever got around to marrying and fathering children, it would have been out of a sense of duty.

This reading should provide a salutary lesson for all overpowering mothers and maiden aunts!

COMMENTARY ON THE READING

The emphasis on an inhibiting mother–son relationship was something of a mystery and certainly the *Dictionary of National Biography*[4] gives no clues—only:

1769   Born
1784   Education at Eton, Brussels (15 years old)
1789   Angers Military Academy (17 years old)
1787   Lieutenant of Foot (18 years old)

It is known that from an early age he was taunted by his older brother as having a different father from the elder brothers, and also that he had a stern and unloving governess. However, if this is the female dominance in his early life, graphology makes too much of it. Comments about his integrity are obviously true and a successful Commander in Chief of a field army must have been able to keep his feelings under control, especially in the heat of battle. He may well have been self-opinionated and his marriage was not a great success. He died aged 81 years old from heart failure.

REFERENCES
[1] Hattersley R 1974 *Nelson* (London: Weidenfeld & Nicholson)
[2] The *Times* 1 October 1984 'Shakespeare tops the autograph price list'
[3] *Encyclopaedia Britannica*
[4] *Dictionary of National Biography*, The Concise Dictionary, Part 1, from the beginning to 1900 (Oxford: Oxford University Press)

Finger Reckoning in the Middle Ages

One of the few Europeans who did enough in mathematics during the Middle Ages to be remembered today was Leonardo of Pisa (1175–1230) also known as Fibonacci, who wrote *A Book of Counting* in 1202. He described three methods of solving problems, one involving Arabic numerals, one the abacus and the third, finger reckoning. The people of the Middle Ages went in for the latter in a big way, and indeed, solving problems with fingers goes back far beyond the Middle Ages and it is not now generally realised that big numbers could be represented on the fingers. There was a system of finger signs in the same way that there is a system using hand signals for the deaf.

A person could also multiply with his or her fingers, and with finger reckoning one would only need to know one's multiplication tables up to 5 × 5.

Here is how one would do 6 × 9 on one's fingers: On one hand hold up one finger (the difference between the five fingers on that hand and

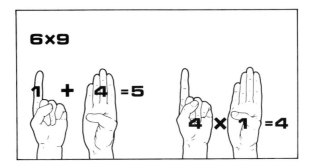

6×9

1 + 4 =5

4 × 1 =4

Add *the* standing fingers *to get the* tens *and* multiply *the* closed fingers *to get the* units.

the first of the numbers to be multiplied, i.e. six). On the other hand hold up four fingers, the difference between five and nine. Then *add* the standing fingers (1 + 4 = 5) to get the tens of the answer. In this case there would be five tens, so one would know that the answer would be 50-something. To find the 'something' *multiply* the closed fingers (4 × 1 = 4), thus reaching the answer of 54. A similar system could be used to multiply numbers between 10 and 15. Take the problem 14 × 12. Put up four fingers on one hand and two on the other. Add them to get six; then add 10 times that sum to 100, which would give you 160; finally add the product of the fingers, 4 × 2, to reach the answer: 168. If you know algebra the equation: $xy = 10\ [(x - 10) + (y - 10)] + 100 + (x - 10)(y - 10)$ will show you why this system works.

REFERENCE
Adapted from Rogers J T 1968 *The Story of Mathematics* (Leicester: Brockhampton Press)

Metoposcopy: Observation of the Forehead

The great exponent of metoposcopy was Jerome Cardan, a polymath whose many activities included medicine, astronomy, mathematics, astrology and the occult arts. He was born in 1500, the illegitimate son of a Milanese scholar who was both a doctor in medicine and law and also a competent mathematician. Jerome's education was rather irregular but, among other subjects, he studied medicine as well as mathematics and music and received an MD degree from Padua in 1526. He was an inveterate gambler, obstinate and cantankerous, and made many enemies. However, although his life was full of mis-

148

fortune, he achieved great fame as an astrologer as well as a physician and travelled to Paris, London and Edinburgh to practice astrology and medicine. It was in London in 1552 that he cast the horoscope of King Edward VI, the son and successor of King Henry VIII. Cardan's predictions, though, were abysmally wrong and he foretold that Edward would live at least until his 55th birthday and then suffer from various diseases. In fact, he died in 1553 before reaching his 17th birthday. The excuse by Cardan, given in King (1973), is:

> It was unsafe to pronounce upon the term of life in weak nativities, unless all processes, and ingresses, and external movement that from month to month and year to year affect the ruling planets had been carefully inquired into. But to make such a calculation would have cost him, he said, not less than a hundred hours.

and then apparently he added a few more reasons!

Cardan, when he presented the subject of metoposcopy, reminds us of some present day writers on palmistry. First, he provided some blanket statements that could serve as excuses-in-advance. Metoposcopy, he said is an art, but like navigation, agriculture or medicine, it is by no means infallible. By regarding the lines on the forehead and the configuration of the head, we cannot really have complete confidence in the future, but we can predict what will happen *for the most part*. Knowledge is increased as we take into account other factors, including parents, education, age, palmistry and the constitution of the stars. Using all this information, we can make fairly safe judgements.

To indicate the validity of metoposcopy, Cardan cited a case from Suetonius, from the life of Titus. A person skilled in metoposcopy correctly predicted that Britannicus, the son of the Emperor Claudius, would not ascend the throne, but that Titus, then a child, would do so. This type of citation is of course a familiar method of *proving* the validity of prophecy by pointing to a particular case where a prediction came true. Cardan bolstered this argument by claiming that we never find a wicked man who entirely lacks the signs of wickedness on his forehead, but no upright person is contaminated by these signs.

He presented various rules that seemed to govern the art of metoposcopy and distinguished seven horizontal lines in the forehead each correlated with a different planet. This was necessary since the planets and the zodiac are central in all divinatory arts.

In addition to the major horizontal lines, there are others that intersect, forming small figures such as crosses, circles, squares, triangles and stellate figures, each having its own significance. Lines are to be judged by various qualities: if continuous, they indicate good fortune; if interrupted, adversity of some type; if prominent, they

149

Cardans's map of the forehead, indicating the spheres of influence of the planets.

signify great and noteworthy events or a manifest effect of the planet represented; but if small or delicate, then obscure events or feeble effects. Curving lines reveal an exaltation that subsides. Branching lines mean trouble. When crossed, they portend danger and harm from the planet represented. The major lines are divisible into three portions: the left third have to do with early life, up to age 30; the middle third to age 60; and the right side to old age, approximately 90. Lines that ascend to the right are favourable, those that descend are bad.

Furthermore, various other marks on the forehead or face, such as naevi, have a significance of their own and may change the interpretation. Just as the lines on the forehead are associated with the planets, so are the various naevi on the face.

Cardan presented a large number of individual case reports with diagrammatic reproductions of the facial ines and marks, together with a brief forecast. But he did not link up his individual cases with general principles and hence there is no way to see how he derived his

150

prophecies. Nor was there any follow-up to say if the predictions were valid!

Examples of case reports are:

The *man who is marked with these lines will die of plague.*

This man will die of bladder stone.

The *three semicircular lines with two straight ones, and a naevus on the right cheek, promises him a long life and great honour outside his country.*

This is the forehead of an unfortunate woman. The lines in the form of a cross denote a woman corrupted before and after her marriage, who nevertheless will have two husbands. The naevus here against the right zygoma means that she will have intercourse (commercium) *with churchmen* (ecclesiasticus) *and will die of poison.*

Unlike palmistry, metoposcopy and the more obscure forms of prediction have fallen on hard times and are largely forgotten, except for one notable reference in the *Journal of the American Medical Association* in August 1968 (**205** 470). In this article, the authors noted a correlation between certain lines in the forehead (the vertical furrows between the eyebrows) and the coexistence of chronic duodenal ulcers. In a single-blind study they showed in one series that 87% of their patients with ulcer had three or more vertical furrows, but only 5% of the control patients with no ulcer were in this metoposcopical group. Their study presented the graphical distribution of vertical forehead lines in 400 patients and those with ulcers seemed significantly separated from the controls. However, it must be emphasised that these authors gave their explanations in terms of modern medical science—the planets were ignored!

REFERENCES

Text adapted from King L S 1973 'Metoposcopy and kindred arts' *J. Am. Med. Assoc.* **224** 42–6

Illustrations from 1658 *Metoposcopia* (Paris: Thomas Jolly)

Charms against Teething

Shown below is a charm against teething consisting of a necklet of small shells. It was used in Jersey.

One of the most common charms for teething was the orris root, used in Norfolk and east London among other places, but there were

Left: *Necklet of shells from Seville.* Right: *Orris root, which was used not only in England but was also rubbed on the gums of Jewish children in the Balkan States and in Poland. (Courtesy Wellcome Institute Library, London.)*

also pigs' feet (south London), a necklet of nightshade (Gloucestershire and Warwickshire), calves' teeth (south London), a pimento necklace (Yorkshire), a bag of split ash twigs (Devon) and a wolf's tooth worn on a cap not only to guard against teething troubles but also to avert evil spirits (Palestine).

Charm against Nightmares

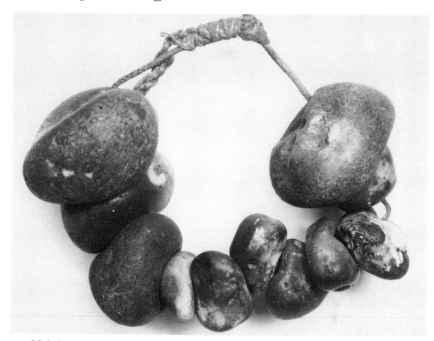

Holed stones to be hung at the head of the bed as a charm against nightmares. (Courtesy Wellcome Institute Library, London.)

Rabbit Fights Back

Natural justice, but not the police, has caught up with two men in South Australia who killed a rabbit with high explosive. According to a free magazine distributed to Australian expatriates in London, police are looking for the two who apparently tied a stick of gelignite to the bunny and lit the fuse before setting the terrified animal free. 'The trick backfired,' the magazine reports, 'when the rabbit took cover under their four-wheel drive vehicle. The men escaped but their $20 000 utility was wrecked.'

REFERENCE
New Scientist 16 August 1984 p. 41

Charm against Rheumatism

This amulet against rheumatism was two mole's feet in a satchel. (From Sussex, England.) Mole's feet were also used as a charm for toothache in Norfolk, an alternative in Wiltshire was joined hazel-nuts and in Devon, stones or teeth. (Courtesy Wellcome Institute Library, London.)

154

Suicide

A monologue written by Roy Clegg and Harold Clegg-Walker in 1931.

Now I am a fellow who's lived—
    I've lived and I've loved and I've lost,
I loved a fair damsel who didn't love me,
    So my fate to the winds must be tossed.
She laughed when I tried to be serious,
    Her pretty heels trampled my heart,
The future means nothing, so now I must die,
    But the question is—how do I start?
To jump in a river and drown
    Is a good plan, or so I've been told.
But if some poor simpleton does fish you out,
    You get such a terrible cold.
To turn on the gas and be smothered
    Is one way, but you never can tell
If someone will biff in and spoil the whole thing,
    And just curse you for making a smell.
To hang by the neck on one's braces
    Is sometimes considered the thing,
But I fear mine would hardly stand up to the strain,
    For already they're tied up with string.
I like the idea of revolvers,
    I'd prefer to be shot than to hang,
But ever since childhood I've always been scared
    Of things that go off with a bang.
I once had a vague sort of notion
    Of leaping beneath an express,
But one has to consider one's fellows, you know,
    The chappies who clear up the mess.
Still the Underground might offer scope,
    One could sit down upon a live rail,
But that involves trespassing—what a disgrace
    If the corpse had to serve time in jail.
Now Keatings kills bugs, moths and beetles,
    In that case it ought to kill me.
The butler must make me some sandwiches, James!
    No. Dash it! he's gone out to tea.
Never mind though, there must be some way,
    Such as hurling yourself from a cliff,
Even then you might find that you'd only been
        stunned,
    And you'd wake up most frightfully stiff.

I've given up thinking of razors,
   I've tried and I'm wondering yet
How those fellows who do it can cut their own throats,
   It's a thing beyond my Gillette.
No, really, I'm finding that this sort of thing's
   Not as easily done as it's said.
So I think I'll pop off for the week-end or so—
   And perhaps shoot some rabbits instead.

REFERENCE

Marshall M (ed) 1981 *The Book of Comic and Dramatic Monologues* (London: Elm Tree Books/EMI Publishing). Reproduced by permission of EMI Music Publishing Ltd.

Anointing

It may come as a surprise to many that the anointing is no inconsiderable part of the coronation service; but so it is, and it would even be correct to describe it as more important than the crowning itself—more important, that is, from the inner and significant aspect of the ceremony. As part of the coronation ritual anointing was introduced into England in 871, when King Alfred came to the throne, and into Scotland in 1097, when King Edgar was crowned; it now forms a culminating point in the solemn spectacle enacted in Westminster Abbey, when a new monarch comes to rule as King of the United Kingdom of Great Britain and Ireland and of the British Dominions beyond the seas. It is interesting, further, to recollect that anointing has a long history behind it, and that it probably took origin, as A E Crawley asserts [*Encyclopaedia of Religion and Ethics* 1908 vol. 1 pp 549–57], in pre-theistic and even pre-fetish times. At first unguents, varying in nature from a crude animal fat to a perfumed vegetable oil, were used for cosmetic purposes; they gave to the body, after bathing, a feeling of comfort and they were useful in hot climates to protect the skin against the sun's rays and in cold countries to prevent the escape of the body heat. But soon a new meaning—the aesthetic—was added to the cosmetic; the oil gave a gloss to the skin, and the effect was increased by the admixture of a colouring substance. 'Of the majority of early peoples,' says Crawley, 'it may be said that grease and ochre constitute their wardrobe.' In this way personal attractiveness was sought for, and, in the opinion of those interested, was obtained. What, then, could be more natural than to anoint the

156

body for such special occasions as festivals and holy days? The honoured guest also was welcomed with bathing and anointing, and inanimate objects were polished and to some extent preserved from decay by being rubbed with unguents. It is easy to link on these uses to the magical and religious employment of ointments, but in the process a new notion is found to have come in. Organic matter is believed to be instinct with some Divine force or vital essence and to have a magical or supernatural power; further, this power can be transmitted either by eating and drinking the specially sacred matter, or, more easily and doubtless more safely, by external application of it to the body of the worshipper. Fat has come to occupy a curiously important place among the substances which are held to transmit the desirable gifts of life and strength; and it is reported, for instance; that the Australian savage will kill a man to get his kidney fat for anointing himself with. A further stage in development sees fat consecrated in various ways, so that it may serve as the vehicle for the transmission of a Divine Essence. It can now be seen how anointing has entered into medical practice, not by one, but by several routes. There has been the belief in the magical effect of the fat as well as in the sacred influence which it carries; there has been in an interesting way (too intricate to enter into here) the principle of the removal of tabu; there has been the discovery of the invigorating effect of rubbing the skin with oil; and there has been the knowledge of the action of the unguent upon the cutaneous secretions and upon transpiration. If to these be added the ascertained therapeutic effects of various medicinal substances, we are possessed of a series of contributing causes which sufficed to introduce anointing into medicine and to keep it among the accredited means of treating disease.'

REFERENCE
Br. Med. J. 1911 **1** 1479–80 (published at the time of the coronation of King George V)

Leonardo's Last Supper

A most bizarre representation of the Leonardo masterpiece in the Sistine Chapel in the Vatican—on the back of Mrs Emma de Burgh of the USA. Nineteenth century photograph in the publication *La*

Nature. The tatoos were executed by the Riley brothers on the husband and wife Frank and Emma de Burgh.

(Courtesy Mary Evans Picture Library.)

(*Courtesy Mary Evans Picture Library.*)

The Royal Wedding

The following is an extract from a young schoolgirl's essay on the wedding of Prince Charles and Lady Diana Spencer. It was first overheard in 1982 as part of an after-dinner speech by an eminent

Archdeacon—*and is true.*

. . . Prince Charles rode in an open cart, but Dinah and Father Earl Spencer went by First Class Carriage. As the bride walked the red mat in St. Paul's we saw her veil was held to her head by the Spencer Terror . . .

When the Prince and his Lady had exchanged vowels and the ring was put on to make man and wife, the marriage was consummated in front of the high altar by the Archbishop of Canterbury followed by several of London's top clergy . . .

After the ride back, the Prince and She waves from Buck and Ham Palace from the garage roof . . .

Treatment of Political Prisoners Under a Liberal Government

A suffragette poster, circa 1910, published by the Women's Social and Political Union. (Courtesy Mary Evans Picture Library.)

How Diet Changes Your Personality

The changes in personality which can be caused by strict diets have been given considerable publicity in the last few days following the sentencing of champion racing jockey Lester Piggott for tax evasion

160

on Friday. Piggott virtually starved himself for 30 years to stay at 8st 3lbs—two stones below his normal body weight—and it is thought that his diet might have led to his obsession with hoarding money.

A different effect is reported in the current issue of the *British Medical Journal* which tells the tale of a 68-year-old man who was admitted to hospital after his family had complained that his behaviour had changed dramatically.

This man's normal manner was quiet and reserved, but in his new guise he became over-excited and sleepless. When a doctor visited his home he was racing round non-stop, stark naked, and cracking jokes.

A month before this change, the man had consulted another doctor about heart problems, and had been put on a strict diet of two pints of milk a day with nothing else, to control a rise in his blood pressure.

Once in hospital, tests revealed that the diet had triggered his thyroid gland into over-drive, which in turn had led to his manic behaviour.

Within a month of being taken off the diet, his behaviour had returned to normal.

REFERENCE
The *Independent* 27 October 1987

Medical English

The journal *World Medicine*, which sadly ceased publication in 1984, was well known as a source of anecdotal material. This included regular snippets from the papers and from communications between doctors, patients and hospitals. This is a selection from the years 1977–84.

The condomned murderer and his girlfriend took overdoses today in an apparent suicide pact.

Glasgow Herald

The operation was carried out by a Scot, as was the anaesthetist.

Sunday Post

From our records, we know that 17 patients are using a mechanical method, though this may be the tip of the iceberg.

Health Bulletin

161

My doctor wants me to have the baby in hospital because I'm an elderly primate.

Patient in Sidmouth

I don't wish to be put on the duty rooster at the chicken factory.

Lady patient in Sussex

Lost: green silk umbrella belonging to lady with one broken rib and curiously shaped ivory head.

Herts Advertiser

We shall be at the Curragh for the annual orgasm of the Hospitals' Trust Derby. Of course it is going to be a most gorgeous afternoon . . .

Dublin Evening Press

Thank you for sending this woman along. I have started the bull rolling by requesting a semen analysis.

Letter from infertility clinic, Hertfordshire

Although suicide by a shot in the neck was atypical, the experts said, there were a number of references in scientific literature which described it as a safe method.

The Guardian

Hand painted pub signs could be on their way back in the North West. More than 350 artists submitted entries when a Warrington based brewery invited people to be hung outside their pubs.

Glazebury Journal

Reminiscing about Empire Days past, she told the Policy & Resources Committee: 'In the morning we saluted the flag, and in the afternoon we had it off'.

Worthing Gazette

Impotence as a presenting symptom in this condition is said to be very uncommon, but there is very little hard data.

British Journal of Sexual Medicine

British babies like children casserole best.

The Times

Some men are so disturbed and depressed on receiving a life sentence that they end up getting physiotherapy.

Medical News

Event Nine: The Norden Trophy for the cow with the best udder. Presented by Mr Norden in memory of Mrs Norden.

Guernsey Agricultural Show brochure

Dear Doctor, Could you please leave a note to cover me, as I went into hospital for a scrap on Friday, and to be quarterized.

Note from an Essex patient

Using the embassy diplomatic bog to smuggle weapons and ammunition into Britain.

Daily Telegraph

Dear Doctor, Please come quickly—diarrhoea very bad and going downhill rapidly.

Request for visit, Edinburgh

The hospital's new diagnostic services include three x-ray rooms and nine extra places in the mortuary.

Ormskirk Advertiser

Two hundred and twenty three patients have been waiting for gynaecological surgery on their ears, nose or throat.

Manchester Evening News

The unusual series of sex change operations involves a bilateral mastectomy, hysterectomy and penal surgery.

Aberdeen Evening Express

Wanted: Assistant or associate professor in plastic, reconstructive and bum surgery.

University of Kuwait advertisment

An American surgeon lecturing medical students in Bristol was asked if he considered the operation he was describing was a valuable one. 'Valuable' demanded the surgeon, a little taken aback. 'I raised five kids on it'.

Financial Times

I saw this patient of yours in the clinic. She does appear to be pregnant, and there are social difficulties, with the possibility of the child not being hers.

Note from Manchester obstetrician

Quack Chinese doctors are paying £40 000 for bodies snatched from graves. They use parts of the bodies to make medicines that guarantee immortality.

Yorkshire Evening Post

For Sale: Rolls Royce hearse, with 1965 body.

Droitwich Gazette

Members of the family request mourners to omit floral tributes. The deceased was allergic to flowers.

New York obituary column

Throwing caution to the wind, I ordered a tournedos and half a giraffe of wine.

Manchester Evening News

The patient changed to Guinness under the mistaken belief that it would not affect his lever.

Surrey consultant's letter

Come to enjoy us in our spectacular LA HACIENDA with mariachis, music, beautiful open terrace and air conditioned entrails. Nice. Clean.

Acapulco Hotel News

Nuclear Leak. The underground control centre to be used at Kettering, Northants, in the event of a nuclear attack, has only an outside lavatory, according to a report to be considered by county councillors.

Daily Telegraph

Gallstones go with a bang. Doctors at a hospital in the ancient Chinese capital of Xian have perfected a new way of disposing of gall bladder stones. They blow them up with micro-explosives. Physicians insert an apparatus into the bladder, bore a hole in the stone, insert tiny explosives and reduce the stone to fragments which are discharged in the urine.

Xinhua: official Chinese news agency

Even the post mortem failed to establish a precise diagnosis and no useful treatment was subsequently initiated.

Hospital Doctor

When the Bull Beats the Matador

The *British Medical Journal* of 12 July 1986 carried the following item previously reported in the *Journal of the Royal Society of Medicine* concerning a conference in Spain.

A Spanish surgeon who contributed to the meeting included several bullfight injuries in his series of patients with traumatic lesions of the anal sphincter. Apparently only cowardly matadors come to the proctologist; the brave full frontal ones are said to provide business for the urologists.

164

The Many Pains of Snoring

Heavy snoring may sometimes be a sign of serious heart disease, but it can also lead to other unexpected painful conditions, as described in a letter in the *New England Journal of Medicine*.

A 66-year-old man from Toronto consulted his GP about a dull pain deep in the muscle of his calf. The GP could not find any major abnormalities, prescribed pain-killers and suggested the man return if the pain intensified.

Two nights later, the patient had just fallen asleep when he was abruptly awoken by a sharp pain in the same calf, the result of a kick by his wife. His remonstration: 'Don't kick me there, that's just where my leg hurts,' was greeted with the reply: 'You were snoring again, and that's where I always kick you to stop it.'

After some discussion his wife agreed to stop kicking. Unfortunately, he could not keep his side of the bargain and continued snoring, but the pain in his calf disappeared within three days.

REFERENCE
The *Independent* 6 October 1987

A Student's Criminals

The statistical significance test, often used in medicine, is a test of the difference between two mean values. The *t*-distribution which under-lies the test was discovered in 1908 by W S Gosset, who was a brewer working for the Guinness Company. The data which he studied for the *t*-distribution came from records of the heights of 3000 criminals. Gosset, who published under the pseudonym 'student', took 750 samples, each of the heights of four criminals, and used these data to calculate 750 means.

REFERENCE
Mould R F 1989 *Introductory Medical Statistics* 2nd edn (Bristol: Hilger)

An Old-Time Apothecary

This figure of the apothecary with his pestle and mortar forms one of the details in the choir of Amiens Cathedral, and since these date from 1508–19 this representation of a pharmacist is from about the time of the Field of the Cloth of Gold.

REFERENCE
The Chemist & Druggist 4 September 1920 (*Courtesy Wellcome Institute Library, London.*)

The Aetiology and Treatment of Childhood[1,2]

This paper originally appeared in the *Journal of Polymorphous Perversity* 1985 **2** 3–7. © Wry-Bred Press Inc. 1985

Childhood is a syndrome which has only recently begun to receive serious attention from clinicians. The syndrome itself, however, is not at all recent. As early as the eighth century, the Persian historian Kidnom made reference to 'short, noisy creatures,' who may well have been what we now call 'children.' The treatment of children, however, was unknown until this century, when so-called 'child psychologists' and 'child psychiatrists' became common. Despite this history of clinical neglect, it has been estimated that well over half of all Americans alive today have experienced childhood directly (Suess 1983). In fact, the actual numbers are probably much higher, since these data are based on self-reports which may be subject to social desirability biases and retrospective distortion.

The growing acceptance of childhood as a distinct phenomenon is reflected in the proposed inclusion of the syndrome in the upcoming *Diagnostic and Statistical Manual of Mental Disorders, 4th Edition,* or *DSM-IV*, of the American Psychiatric Association (1985). Clinicians are still in disagreement about the significant clinical features of childhood, but the proposed *DSM-IV* will almost certainly include the following core features:

1. Congenital onset
2. Dwarfism
3. Emotional lability and immaturity
4. Knowledge deficits
5. Legume anorexia

CLINICAL FEATURES OF CHILDHOOD

Although the focus of this paper is on the efficacy of conventional treatment of childhood, the five clinical markers mentioned above merit further discussion for those unfamiliar with this patient population.

---

[1] The author would like to thank all the little people.
[2] This research was funded in part by a grant from Bazooka Gum.

Congenital onset. In one of the few existing literature reviews on childhood, Temple-Black (1982) has noted that childhood is almost always present at birth, although it may go undetected for years or even remain subclinical indefinitely. This observation has led some investigators to speculate on a biological contribution to childhood. As one psychologist has put it, 'we may soon be in a position to distinguish organic childhood from functional childhood' (Rogers 1979).

Dwarfism. This is certainly the most familiar clinical marker of childhood. It is widely known that children are physically short relative to the population at large. Indeed, common clinical wisdom suggests that the treatment of the so-called 'small child' (or 'tot') is particularly difficult. These children are known to exhibit infantile behaviour and display a startling lack of insight (Tom and Jerry 1967).

Emotional lability and immaturity. This aspect of childhood is often the only basis for a clinician's diagnosis. As a result, many otherwise normal adults are misdiagnosed as children and must suffer the unnecessary social stigma of being labelled a 'child' by professionals and friends alike.

Knowledge deficits. While many children have IQs within or even above the norm, almost all will manifest knowledge deficits. Anyone who has known a real child has experienced the frustration of trying to discuss any topic that requires some general knowledge. Children seem to have little knowledge about the world they live in. Politics, art and science—children are largely ignorant of these. Perhaps it is because of this ignorance, but the sad fact is that most children have few friends who are not, themselves, children.

Legume anorexia. This last identifying feature is perhaps the most unexpected. Folk wisdom is supported by empirical observation—children will rarely eat their vegetables (see Popeye 1957, for review).

CAUSES OF CHILDHOOD

Now that we know what it is, what can we say about the causes of childhood? Recent years have seen a flurry of theory and speculation from a number of perspectives. Some of the most prominent are reviewed below.

Sociological model. Emile Durkind was perhaps the first to speculate about sociological causes of childhood. He points out two key observations about children: 1) the vast majority of children are unemployed, and 2) children represent one of the least educated segments of our society. In fact, it has been estimated that less than 20% of children have had more than a fourth grade education.

168

Clearly, children are an 'out-group.' Because of their intellectual handicap, children are even denied the right to vote. From the sociologist's perspective, treatment should be aimed at helping assimilate children into mainstream society. Unfortunately, some victims are so incapacitated by their childhood that they are simply not competent to work. One promising rehabilitation program (Spanky and Alfalfa 1978) has trained victims of severe childhood to sell lemonade.

Biological model. The observation that childhood is usually present from birth has led some to speculate on a biological contribution. An early investigation by Flintstone and Jetson (1939) indicated that childhood runs in families. Their survey of over 8000 American families revealed that over half contained more than one child. Further investigation revealed that even most non-child family members had experienced childhood at some point. Cross-cultural studies (e.g. Mowgli and Din 1950) indicate that familial childhood is even more prevalent in the Far East. For example, in Indian and Chinese families, as many as three out of four family members may have childhood.

Impressive evidence of a genetic component of childhood comes from a large scale twin study by Brady and Partridge (1972). These authors studied over 106 pairs of twins, looking at concordance rates for childhood. Among identical or monozygotic twins, concordance was unusually high (0.92), i.e. when one twin was diagnosed with childhood, the other twin was almost always a child as well.

Psychological models. A considerable number of psychologically based theories of the development of childhood exist. They are too numerous to review here. Among the more familiar models are Seligman's 'learned childishness' model. According to this model, individuals who are treated like children eventually give up and become children. As a counterpoint to such theories, some experts have claimed that childhood does not really exist. Szasz (1980) has called 'childhood' an expedient label. In seeking conformity, we handicap those whom we find unruly or too short to deal with by labelling them 'children'.

TREATMENT OF CHILDHOOD

Efforts to treat childhood are as old as the syndrome itself. Only in modern times, however, have humane and systematic treatment protocols been applied. In part, this increased attention to the problem may be due to the sheer number of individuals suffering from childhood. Government statistics (DHSS) reveal that there are more children alive today than at any time in our history. To paraphrase P T Barnum: 'There's a child born every minute.'

The overwhelming number of children has made government intervention inevitable. The nineteenth century saw the institution of what remains the largest single programme for the treatment of childhood —so-called 'public schools.' Under this colossal programme, individuals are placed into treatment groups based on the severity of their condition. For example, those most severely afflicted may be placed in a 'kindergarten' programme. Patients at this level are typically short, unruly, emotionally immature, and intellectually deficient. Given this type of individual, therapy is of necessity very basic. The strategy is essentially one of patient management and of helping the child master basic skills (e.g. finger painting).

Unfortunately, the 'school' system has been largely ineffective. Not only is the programme a massive tax burden, but it has failed even to slow down the rising incidence of childhood.

Faced with this failure and the growing epidemic of childhood, mental health professionals are devoting increasing attention to the treatment of childhood. Given a theoretical framework by Freud's landmark treatises on childhood, child psychiatrists and psychologists claimed great successes in their clinical interventions.

By the 1950s, however, the clinicians' optimism had waned. Even after years of costly analysis, many victims remained children. The following case (taken from Gumbie and Pokey 1957) is typical.

> Billy J., age 8, was brought to treatment by his parents. Billy's affliction was painfully obvious. He stood only 4' 3" high and weighed a scant 70 pounds, despite the fact that he ate voraciously. Billy presented a variety of troubling symptoms. His voice was noticeably high for a man. He displayed legume anorexia and, according to his parents, often refused to bathe. His intellectual functioning was also below normal —he had little general knowledge and could barely write a structured sentence. Social skills were also deficient. He often spoke inappropriately and exhibited 'whining behaviour.' His sexual experience was non-existent. Indeed, Billy considered women 'icky.'
>
> His parents reported that his condition had been present from birth, improving gradually after he was placed in a school at age 5. The diagnosis was 'primary childhood'. After years of painstaking treatment, Billy improved gradually. At age 11, his height and weight have increased, his social skills are broader, and he is now functional enough to hold down a 'paper route.'

After years of this kind of frustration, startling new evidence has come to light which suggests that the prognosis in cases of childhood may not be all gloom. A critical review by Fudd (1972) noted that studies of the childhood syndrome tend to lack careful follow-up. Acting on this observation, Moe, Larrie and Kirly (1974) began a large scale longitudinal study. These investigators studied two groups.

The first group comprised 34 children currently engaged in a long-term conventional treatment programme. The second was a group of 42 children receiving no treatment. All subjects had been diagnosed as children at least 4 years previously, with a mean duration of childhood of 6.4 years.

At the end of one year, the results confirmed the clinical wisdom that childhood is a refractory disorder—virtually all symptoms persisted and the treatment group was only slightly better off than the controls.

The results, however, of a careful 10-year follow-up were startling. The investigators (Moe, Larrie, Kirly and Shemp 1984) assessed the original cohort on a variety of measures. General knowledge and emotional maturity were assessed with standard measures. Height was assessed by the 'metric system' (see Ruler 1923), and legume appetite by the Vegetable Appetite Test (VAT) designed by Popeye (1968). Moe et al found that subjects improved uniformly on all measures. Indeed, in most cases, the subjects appeared to be symptom-free. Moe et al report a spontaneous remission rate of 95%, a finding which is certain to revolutionize the clinical approach to childhood.

These recent results suggest that the prognosis for victims of childhood may not be so bad as we have feared. We must not, however, become too complacent. Despite its apparently high spontaneous remission rate, childhood remains one of the most serious and rapidly growing disorders facing mental health professionals today. And, beyond the psychological pain it brings, childhood has recently been linked to a number of physical disorders. Twenty years ago, Howdi, Doody and Beauzeau (1965) demonstrated a six-fold increased risk of chicken pox, measles and mumps among children compared with normal controls. Later, Barby and Kenn (1971) linked childhood to an elevated risk of accidents—compared with normal adults, victims of childhood were much more likely to scrape their knees, lose teeth and fall off their bikes.

Clearly, much more research is needed before we can give any real hope to the millions of victims wracked by this insidious disorder.

REFERENCES

American Psychiatric Association 1985 *The diagnostic and statistical manual of mental disorders, 4th edition: A preliminary report.* (Washington, DC: APA).

Barby B and Kenn K 1971 The plasticity of behavior. In B Barby and K Kenn (eds) *Psycho-therapies R Us* (Detroit: Ronco Press).

Brady C and Partridge S 1972 My dad's bigger than your dad *Acta Eur. Age* **9** 123–6

Flintstone F and Jetson G 1939 Cognitive mediation of labor disputes *Industrial Psychology Today* **2** 23–35

Fudd E J 1972 Locus of control and shoe-size *Journal of Footwear Psychology* **78** 345–56

Gumbie G and Pokey P A cognitive theory of iron smelting *Journal of Abnormal Metallurgy* **45** 235–9

Howdi C, Doodi C and Beauzeau C 1965 Western civilization: A review of the literature *Reader's Digest* **60** 23–5

Moe R, Larrie T and Kirly Q 1974 State childhood vs. trait childhood *TV Guide* May 12–19 1–3

Moe R, Larrie T, Kirly Q and Shemp C 1984 Spontaneous remission of childhood. In W C Fields (ed) *New Hope for Children and Animals* (Hollywood: Acme Press)

Popeye T S M 1957 The use of spinach in extreme circumstances *Journal of Vegetable Science* **58** 530–8

Popeye T S M 1968 Spinach: A phenomenological perspective *Existential Botany* **35** 908–13

Rogers F 1979 *Becoming My Neighbour* (New York: Soft Press)

Ruler Y 1923 Assessing measurement protocols by the multi-method multiple regression index for the psychometric analysis of factorial interaction. *Annals of Boredom* **67** 1190–260

Spanky D and Alfalfa Q 1978 Coping with puberty *Sears Catalogue* 45–6

Suess D R 1983 A psychometric analysis of green eggs with and without ham *Journal of Clinical Cuisine* **245** 567–78

Temple-Black S 1982 Childhood: An ever-so sad disorder *Journal of Precocity* **3** 129–34

Tom C and Jerry M 1967 Human behavior as a model for understanding the rat. In M de Sade (ed) *The Rewards of Punishment* (Paris: Bench Press, 1967)

FURTHER READINGS

Joe G I 1965 Aggressive fantasy as wish fulfillment *Archives of General MacArthur* **5** 23–45

Leary T 1969 Pharmacotherapy for childhood *Annals of Astrological Science* **67** 456–9

Kissoff K G B 1975 Extinction of learned behavior. Paper presented to the Siberian Psychological Association, 38th Annual Meeting, Kamchatka

Smythe C and Barnes T 1979 Behavior therapy prevents tooth decay *Journal of Behavioral Orthodontics* **5** 79–89

Potash S and Hoser B 1980 A failure to replicate the results of Smythe and Barnes *Journal of Dental Psychiatry* **34** 678–80

Smythe C and Barnes T 1980 Your study was poorly done: A reply to Potash and Hoser *Annual Review of Aquatic Psychiatry* **10** 123–56

Potash S and Hoser B 1981 Your mother wears army boots; A further reply to Smythe and Barnes *Achives of Invective Research* **56** 570–8

Smythe C and Barnes T 1982 Embarrassing moments in the sex lives of Potash and Hoser: A further reply *National Enquirer* May 16

An Italian Quack

The few lines of old Italian poetry at the bottom of the picture
translate as:

The man who from acuteness of intellect,
Wishes to make some anatomical investigation,
is a sharp snake,
He shows over and above his obvious absolute power the privilege
of deceiving the world.

(Courtesy Wellcome Institute Library, London.)

173

The snake is a reference to the Greek god of medicine and healing, Asklepios, who as Aesculapius, was introduced into Rome in 293 BC, in the form of a snake, during a pestilence. Mythology has it that Aesculapius was the son of Apollo and was trained as a physician of miraculous powers by Chiron, the most learned of the Centaurs. Once, it was said, to the annoyance of his grandfather Zeus, he restored a dead man to life. Zeus became jealous and at his request, Pluto hurled a thunderbolt at Aesculapius, which ended his life on earth. Mythology also states that Aesculapius was the ship's doctor on the *Argo* when Jason and the Argonauts searched for the Golden Fleece.

REFERENCE
Mitelli G M 1660 *L'arti per Via* (Bologna: Longhi)

Anecdote of Field Marshall Lord Montgomery

(Contributed by Harold Winter.)

Before the end of the 1939–45 war, a staff officer with high political connections was caught with his 'fingers in the till' in a petrol racket in Tripoli, Syria. At the subsequent Court Martial he was reduced to the lowest officer rank, that of Second Lieutenant, and in a note to Military Intelligence, Monty wrote: 'Fit to fart but not to fight'.

A Scene of Mesmeric Therapy

Mesmer was an Austrian, born in 1734 near Lake Constance, who first trained for the priesthood, later changed his mind and studied law at Vienna University, and then finally transferred to medicine, obtaining his degree in 1766 at the age of 32. Early in 1768 he married a rich widow and it was his wife's cousin Francisca Oesterlin on whom he first tried his 'magnetic treatment'. Mesmer described her medical problem in the following terms: 'She was attacked several years before by a convulsive disease, the most troublesome symptoms of which were that blood rushed with impetuosity to the head, and excited in that part agonising pain in the teeth and ears which was followed by delirium, maniacal elatement, vomiting and syncope'.

Mesmer's belief in animal magnetism arose from his MD thesis in which he studied the suupposed influence of the Sun and the Moon on

174

the human body. He believed that they caused an ebb and flow in the body analogous to the tides. His treatment was intended to restore harmony between the individual and the universe. He treated his patients by fitting magnets to various parts of the body and was able to affect many dramatic 'cures'—but this was in effect an early example of successful psychotherapy, rather than proof of animal magnetism, and more orthodox physicians in Austria were always sceptical.

Eventually, his fate as a physician and magnetiser in Austria was sealed by the outcome of his treatment of Marie-Therese Paradis, a pianist who had been blind since the age of four. Mesmer had restored her eyesight (the problem would now be recognised as hysterical blindness). Her father was a secretary to the Emperor of Austria and was afraid that his daughter's pension and other advantages might now be forfeit. His attitude caused his daughter to relapse into her previous state and in the aftermath Mesmer was disgraced and left Vienna for Paris in 1778.

This oil was painted c. 1800 and shows Franz Anton Mesmer holding a wand, right background of the painting. (Courtesy Wellcome Institute Library, London.)

He bcame financially successful in Paris with many patients, and typically he would induce a state of trance by touching them with a wand, and after a short while they would break into a sweat and be siezed by convulsions. Many then threw themselves at his feet in gratitude.

175

However, his popularity made enemies of French physicians and in 1784 King Louis XVI set up a Royal Commission to investigate animal magnetism. Members of the Commission included the then American Ambassador to France, Benjamin Franklin; Joseph Guillotin the inventor of the guillotine; and Antoine Lavoisier the famous chemist. They failed to prove the existence of animal magnetism, and Dr Charles d'Elson (physician to the future King Charles X), Mesmer's most prominent supporter, was expelled from the Paris Medical Faculty. Mesmer was forced to retire, fled through Europe and eventually settled at Meersburg, Switzerland, on Lake Constance, where he died in 1815.

Samuel Butler's Description of the Human Body

A pair of pincers set over a bellow and a stewpan and the whole fixed on stilts.

Anecdote of Sir Clement Price Thomas

Sir Clement Price Thomas was an eminent thoracic surgeon at the Westminster and Brompton Hospitals who was in charge of the lung cancer operation on King George VI. This anecdote concerns a less eminent occasion.

A new firm of medical students had just been appointed to Sir Clement Price Thomas and were standing round the bed of a patient waiting for the great man to arrive. He duly did so, and asked whether certain matters had yet occurred, such as the taking of blood pressure, pulse rate, etc preparatory to making a clinical decision.

'Yes', said the students, meekly.

'Well, what is your decision?' asked Sir Clement.

There was a pause, but no answer.

'Well, would you operate?'

The students were over-awed, but one managed to summon enough courage to reply, decided to be conservative, and said 'No'. The other five, having even less courage, followed suit and also said 'No'.

'But *I* would' said the eminent surgeon, at which point a voice from the bed said in a loud Cockney London accent,

176

'No you won't mate, what, with 6 to 1 against, do you think I'm daft?'.—The patient was a bookmaker!

Lettsom's Moral and Physical Thermometer

LETTSOM'S MORAL AND PHYSICAL THERMOMETER, OR THE SCALE OF THE PROGRESS OF TEMPERANCE AND INTEMPERANCE.

(Courtesy Wellcome Institute Library, London.)

REFERENCE
Abraham J J 1933 *Lettsom* (London: Heinemann) p. 484

Impromptu Speech

How wonderful is the human brain. It starts working before we are born, it continues, waking or sleeping, until the day we die and the only time it stops is when someone asks us to stand up and say a few words.

REFERENCE
Kenny P 1982 *A Handbook of Public Speaking for Scientists and Engineers* (Bristol: Adam Hilger) p. 50

Anecdote of Virchow and Bismarck

The eminent physiologist Rudolf Virchow criticised the German Chancellor Bismarck who challenged him to a duel. Since Virchow was the challenged, he chose the weapons. He held up two large sausages and said 'One contains the germ of trichinosis and the other is harmless. Let his Excellency choose and eat and I will eat the other'. Bismarck decided to laugh off the affront—and the duel.

The Dinner-plate Twins

On Nelson's flagship there were twins, one with dinner-plate ears and one with dinner-plate eyes. The twin with the dinner-plate eyes was always posted to the crow's nest at the top of the tallest mast to look for enemy ships. He spotted one and called down to his Admiral: 'Admiral, there is a French ship three miles away on the horizon'.

Nelson was most impressed but asked how he knew it was a French ship. The reply was: 'My brother overheard them talking'.

Advertisement for a Surgeon–Dentist

(Courtesy Wellcome Institute Library, London.)

Persian Wisdom

The best thing you can bring back from your travel is yourself unscathed.

REFERENCE
Manila Bulletin 12 February 1985

The Pestäule in Vienna

This monument, the Pestäule, is in the Graben in Vienna, near to St Stephen's Cathedral. It commemorates Leopold I's thanksgiving after the plague of April 1679 which took thousands of lives. The column is made of white Salzburg marble surrounded by cloud spirals and crowned by the Trinity in gilded copper. Nine angels in groups of three carry the emblems of Leopold's power, the lance and the Duke's hat, coat of arms and sword, and crown and sceptre. On the bottom part of the monument are the coats of arms of the House of Austria and of the Kingdoms of Hungary and of Bohemia.

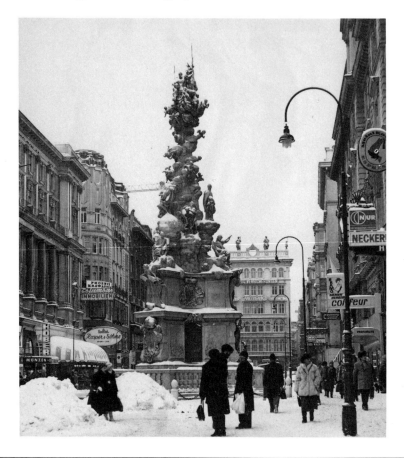

Miraculous Medical Properties of Russian Vodka

Shortly after the Chernobyl accident on 26 April 1986 various newspapers reported that the local population of Kiev, a city of 2.5 million inhabitants some 120 kilometres distant from the Chernobyl nuclear power station, were taking a radiation exposure antidote. This was apparently a mixture of Kiev vodka and strong red wine. The only logical reason for such a theory was presumably that after an adequate dose the patient would be incapable of worrying about nuclear fallout, civil or military!

180

I ignored these accounts as old wives tales until I actually visited the Chernobyl site and its evacuated dormitory town of Pripyat on 2 December 1987. The stories were true. People actually did believe that vodka 'helped'. Indeed, a scientist who should have known better even had a biological theory to justify the 'medicine'. The vodka goes straight to the cells of the body and the radiation always attacks the vodka first rather than any other cellular material and therefore vodka gives a certain amount of protection.

The prescription was: *'Take a bottle of vodka and a bottle of strong red wine. Pour a glass of vodka and add six drops of red wine. Drink. Repeat the prescription until the bottle of red wine is empty.'*.

A medical experiment with mice was also supposed to have been made with one group being given vodka and the control group no vodka. Eventually all were sacrificed for post-mortem studies. No evidence of leukaemia was found in either group, but the vodka-mice had cirrhosis of the liver.

The particular brand of vodka was not specified, but perhaps it was that described to me by Alan Frank of Radio London when my first book of anecdotes was being reviewed. The label is shown below and was originally located in the Bahamas!

100 % NEUTRAL GRAIN SPIRITS
CHARCOAL FILTERED

5238

To Russia with Love!

BOGOROV

БОГОРОВ

100% Pure Vodka

80 PROOF

FIVE TIMES DISTILLED AND FILTERED
THROUGH ACTIVATED CHARCOAL
100 % NEUTRAL GRAIN SPIRITS.

Abortions in Greece, January 1987

As soon as the Chernobyl accident on 26 April 1986 was reported in newspapers and on TV, the actual events (initial deaths at the power plant turned out to be 31: firefighters and plant workers) rapidly became magnified in several countries and guesses by reporters were wildly inaccurate. Thus in the United Kingdom the *Daily Mirror* on 30 April headlined 'Please get me out Mummy', 'Terror of Trapped Britons' and '2,000 are feared dead in Nuclear Horror'. The *Detroit Medical News* of 12 May stated 'So the Russians have started to self-destruct. That is the good news, the bad news is that they are exporting the fallout across the globe.'. The *New York Post* was most outlandish with '15,000 Dead in Mass Grave'. TV was not always much better with an American TV network buying for 20 000 US dollars a video purporting to be Chernobyl burning. Unfortunately for them, the views were recognised by Italians as being those of a fire at a Trieste cement factory. An ABC TV newscaster was reported to have said 'It is one mistake we will try not to make again.'.

The more horrific an accident, the 'better news' it is supposed to make and this will not alter. I even found this attitude when trying to find a publisher for my book *Chernobyl—The Real Story*. I believe that I quite rightly claimed the contents included 'dramatic pictures'. However, one publisher rejected this claim because, as he said, 'there were no pictures of dead bodies with legs and arms missing'.

In the aftermath of this accident at Chernobyl, the panic caused by the incorrect and inadequate available information was particularly poignant in Greece. Pregnant mothers, because of the 'scare', had otherwise wanted pregnancies terminated. The expected number of live births in Greece in January 1987 was some 9000 but in practice, there were only some 7000 live births, a 23% reduction in those expected. This is considered by Greek physicians to be virtually entirely due to the worry concerning the accident and this is corroborated by the number of live births in February and March 1987 being as expected, since for the births expected in these months, relevant information on radiation effects from Chernobyl was available to the Greek physicians and obstetricians.

REFERENCES

R F Mould 1988 *Chernobyl—The Real Story* (Oxford: Pergamon Press Ltd)
D Trichopoulos 1988 Victims of Chernobyl in Greece *British Medical Journal* **295** 1100

Eyewitness Account of the First Physician at the Scene of the Chernobyl Accident, 1986

The following report is, as far as I know, only to be found in the Russian language publication *Youth*, June 1987 issue, and refers to the eyewitness account of the first doctor to arrive at the scene of the accident, Dr Valentin Petrovich Belokon. He was 28 years old at the time of the accident, with two young daughters, Tania aged 5 years and Katya aged $1\frac{1}{2}$ months. He was also a sportsman who specialised in weight lifting and was employed in Pripyat (the nearest town to the power station) as an accident and emergency physician. This interview took place probably some 2 months after the accident and Dr Belokon was again interviewed in the autumn of 1986. He was by then working as a paediatrician in Donetsk and suffered breathing problems as an after-effect of his experiences. The interviewer was a journalist, Yuri Scherbak.

On 25 April 1986 at 2000 hours I started my work in Pripyat, where there is an accident and emergency medical brigade consisting of one physician (myself) and a doctor's assistant, Sasha (Alexander) Ckachok, and six ambulances. On 25 April Sasha and I worked separately and my driver was Anatoly Guymarov. At 0135 on 26 April on my return to the medical centre I was told that there had been a call from the nuclear power plant and that two or three minutes earlier Sasha had left for the power plant. At 0140 he telephoned to say that there was a fire, with several people burnt and that they needed a doctor. I left with my driver and arrived in seven to ten minutes. When we arrived, the guard asked:
   'Why don't you have
   special clothes?'
I did not know they would be needed and was only wearing my doctor's uniform, and since it was an April evening and the night was warm I did not even wear a doctor's cap. I met Kibenok (a fireman lieutenant who later died) and asked:
   'Are there patients
   with burns?'
Kibenok's reply was that:
   'There are no patients with burns but the situation
   is not clear and my boys feel like vomiting.'
My talk with Kibenok was near the energy block (Unit Number 4) where the firemen stood. Pravik (also a fireman lieutenant who later died) and Kibenok had arrived in two cars and Pravik quickly jumped out of the car but did not come to see me. Kzbenok was excited a little and alarmed.

Dr Belokon then described the first of his patients.

Sasha Ckachok had already taken Shashenok (the second power plant worker to die, the first was buried in the rubble of Unit Number 4 whereas Shashenok died of extensive burns) from the nuclear power plant from which he had been pulled by workers after being burnt and crushed by a falling beam. He died on the morning of 26 April in a medical recovery room. The second patient was a young boy about 18 years old. He had vomiting and severe headache, and as I did not yet know about the high level of radiation I asked him:

'What have you eaten and how
did you spend the previous evening?'

His blood pressure at 140 or 150 over 90 was slightly higher than the normal 120 over 80 for an 18 year old. However, the boy was very nervous. At this time, workers who came out of the nuclear power plant were very disturbed and only exclaimed:

'It is horrible.'

and that

'The instruments went off scale.'

Three or four men from the technical staff all had the same symptoms of headache, swollen glands in the neck, dry throat, vomiting and nausea. They all received medication and were then put into a car and sent to Pripyat with my driver Gumarov. After that, several firemen were brought to me and they could not stand on their feet. They were sent to hospital.

The damaged nuclear power plant after the accident (Courtesy: TASS).

Dr Belokon now begins to feel unwell and records that at 1800 on 26 April, many hours after his arrival:

I felt something wrong in my throat and had a headache. Did I understand that it was dangerous? Was I afraid? Yes, I understood. Yes, I was afraid, but when people see a man in a white uniform is near, it makes them quieter. I stood as all of us stood, without any breathing apparatus, without any other means of protection. When it became lighter on 27 April, there was no fire to be seen in the block (Unit Number 4), but there was black smoke and black soot. The reactor was splitting, but not all the time, only as follows: smoke, smoke, then belch. Gumarov arrived back from Pripyat after taking the injured to hospital and I felt weakness in my feet. I did not notice it when I walked, but now it has happened. Gumarov and I waited another five minutes to see if anyone else asked for assistance, but nobody did. That is why I said to the firemen:

'I am going to hospital,
if there is a need, call us again.'

I went home, but before I washed and changed my clothes, I passed iodine to those in the hostel, asked them to close all windows and to keep the children inside. Then I was taken to the treatment department of a hospital by our Dr Diyakanov and given an intravenous infusion. I felt very bad and started to lose my memory, at first partially and then totally. Later, in Moscow, in Clinic No 6, I was in one ward with a dosimetrist. He told me that just after the explosion, all instruments were off-scale, they called to the safety engineer and that engineer answered:

'What is the panic? Where is the shift chief?
When he is available tell him to call me, you
yourself don't panic, such a report (about off-scale
measurements) is not correct.'

REFERENCES
R F Mould 1988 *Chernobyl—The Real Story* (Oxford: Pergamon Press Ltd)
Y Scherbak 1987 *Unost* (June)

Medical Papyri from Egypt

This selection of five papyri show:
1   Care of hands and feet: chiropody.
2   Poliomyelitis: note the thin leg on the left.
3   This was dedicated by Amenhotep to Amon Ra: presumably to cure earache.
4   Effects of famine.
5   A case history of a fracture of the clavicle, *c.* 3000 BC

Examination. If thou examinest a man having a break in his collar bone, thou shouldst find his collar bone short and separated from its fellow.

Diagnosis. Thou shouldst say concerning him 'One having a break in his collar bone. An ailment which I will treat.'

Treatment. Thou shouldst place him prostrate on his back with something folded between his two shoulder blades. Thou shouldst spread out with his two shoulders in order to stretch apart his collar bone until that break falls into its place. Thou shouldst make for him two splints of linen and thou shouldst apply one of them both on the inside of his upper arm and the other the underside of his upper arm. Thou shouldst bind it with YMRW. Treat it afterwards with honey everyday until he recovers.

Other case histories *c.* 3000 BC include fracture of the skull, a wound in the head, a slit in the outer ear, a dislocation of the mandible, dislocation of the cervical vertebra and breast abscess.

1

2

3

4

5

Most-sought-after Plant

The malunggay plant has become a most-sought-after vegetable. Its pods, flowers, leaves and twigs contain 75 calories of food energy, 6 grams protein, 13 grams carbohydrates and 353 milligrams of calcium per 100 grams edible portion. It has more niacin, thiamine, phosphorous and ascorbic acid than other vegetables, and contains an iron compound that helps prevent anaemia.

REFERENCE
The *Manila Bulletin* 11 February 1985

Manioc is a Root of Good and Evil for the Third World

'A day without manioc is like a day without sunshine,' says Richard Brown, an American who works for Zaire's health ministry.

Maybe so, but manioc has its cloudy side, too.

Also known as cassava and a slew of other aliases, manioc is a scraggly looking plant with elephantine starchy roots. It grows in tropical lands and has many uses.

In Europe, manioc is fed to cattle. In the US, it is turned into tapioca pudding. In Brazil, it is put into cars' gasoline tanks in the form of methanol. In parts of Africa, it is used to starch shirts, roof houses and stiffen leather sheaths.

But above all, manioc gets eaten. Five hundred million people in Africa, Latin America and parts of Asia eat it every day, sometimes two or three times a day. It is one of the world's staple foods, the potato of the Third World.

With drought afflicting more than 20 countries in Africa, manioc's importance in Africans' diet is growing. The plant can live on 50 centimetres of rain a year and survive prolonged dry spells after other crops have perished. For Africa's hungry, its roots are an important source of calories. Many Africans grow manioc, and those who don't can buy it for very little.

As with most good things in the Third World, there are catches. The Food and Agriculture Organization notes that manioc 'isn't a balanced food, consisting, as it does, largely of starch.' It 'compares very poorly in vitamins' with other staples, the FAO says.

Manioc rates especially poorly in protein. Nutritionists say that a child can't consume enough manioc alone to avoid severe protein deficiency.

Also, hardy though it may be, manioc can't survive the kind of drought that much of Africa now is experiencing. Another thing: raw manioc contains lethal amounts of cyanide. But it isn't hard to remove most of the poison.

On the dinner plate, manioc looks thick and mushy, and it tastes the same way. Even some of its fans concede that its taste isn't sublime.

'It has no real taste of its own,' says William O Jones, a professor at Stanford University's Food Research Institute and the author of the 1959 book *Manioc in Africa*.

In North America, manioc, despite its use in tapioca pudding, is unlikely to gain fad-food status akin to that of tofu or kiwi. Goya Foods Inc., a New York food wholesaler, sells processed, sliced and frozen yuca—another name for manioc—imported from Costa Rica. It also sells a dry cassava bread imported from the Dominician Republic.

But Conrad Colon, the purchasing agent for Goya, says manioc has a limited market in the US outside Brazilian and Cuban restaurants. 'It's nothing that people go crazy over,' he says.

Most Westerners prefer their manioc fried, if at all. Many Africans like it ground up as a kind of porridge or in cakes or as a moist substitute for rice: you just pound the peeled manioc into a lumpy flour, boil it in water, pour off the excess water and allow the manioc to sit and absorb moisture. Then, if you like, you can pour a meat or a vegetable dish over the manioc.

'If you are organized, you have a pot of manioc flour soaking in reserve all the time and you just change the water once in a while,' says Musa Joh, an accounting student from Gambia who helps manage the Calabash Restaurant in London's African Centre.

Stanford's Mr Jones says it is the ideal dish for the busy bachelor. Just toss the mix in boiling water for a while and eat.

As for cyanide, it takes only about 50 to 60 milligrams of it to kill an adult. 'Bitter' manioc plants contain an average of 200 to 300 milligrams of cyanide in the form of prussic acid in every kilogram of manioc. So-called sweet strains of the plant contain 70 milligrams of cyanide per kilogram.

Traditional methods of preparing manioc by soaking it, peeling it and drying it in the sun get most of the cyanide out. Medical researchers have nonetheless linked chronic cyanide poisoning from residual prussic acid in manioc to a variety of diseases, including cretinism, optic neuritis, liver degeneration and skin problems.

Some scientists believe that manioc may have been the root of the trouble on Henry Morton Stanley's 1887–9 expedition to Africa, during which nearly half of his 600 porters died. Many of the men, who came from parts of Africa where manioc wasn't well-known, unsuspectingly munched raw manioc and keeled over.

But years before that, Stanley was already griping about the food. He said the 'unvarying slices' of manioc 'deserve three-quarters of the blame now lavished on "murderous Africa".'

But the plant remains a popular crop in the Third World. Originally found in Latin America, it was carried around the world by Portuguese colonists. It can be cultivated to heights ranging from 1.5 metres to 3.5 metres and requires almost no care. It is edible from head to toe: roots, stems and leaves.

'It is an extremely cheap source of calories, it is drought resistant and relatively easy to take care of,' says Stanford's Mr Jones.

Stick a 15-centimetre piece of stem in the ground, and a new plant will sprout up. Manioc grows in bad soil, resists pests, and thrives at altitudes ranging from sea level to nearly 2000 metres.

It can be harvested at any time of the year, but it spoils quickly once harvested and develops brown fibrous streaks and freckles. For this reason importers of manioc in Europe or the US run high risks if they can't sell the stuff fast. Britain's main manioc importer failed last year.

What does the future hold for manioc?

The US Agency for International Development is experimenting in Zaire with a new, fast-growing, low-cyanide hybrid of manioc called Pronam F100. The new breed produces 50% more manioc and doesn't require soaking to remove the cyanide.

But Zairian health officials still advise soaking it just in case: 'Some of the old stuff just might slip in.'

It may be safer, but unfortunately Pronam F100 has pretty much the same taste as the manioc eaten by Stanley when he went to find Livingstone in 1871. On that trip he said manioc 'is insipid food for breakfast and dinner throughout a term of three years. A few months and this diet makes the European sigh for his petit verre, caviar, mock-turtle, salmon—with sauce Hollandaise.'

He added that 'British paupers and Sing Sing convicts might fare better.'

REFERENCE
The *Asian Wall Street Journal* 12 February 1985

Charlatan Extracting Teeth

An engraving by Theodor Rombouts. (Courtesy Wellcome Institute Library, London.)

His First Operation: A Short Story by Sir Arthur Conan Doyle

Sir Arthur Conan Doyle was a medical student in Edinburgh from

1876–81 and this story is about a young student's initiation in the rites of surgery.

It was the first day of a winter session, and the third year's man was walking with the first year's man. Twelve o'clock just booming out from the Tron Church.

'Let me see,' said the third year's man, 'you have never seen an operation?'

'Never.'

'Then this way, please. This is Rutherford's historic bar. A glass of sherry, please, for this gentleman. You are rather sensitive, are you not?'

'My nerves are not very strong, I am afraid.'

'Hum! Another glasss of sherry for this gentleman. We are going to an operation now, you know.'

The novice squared his shoulders and made a gallant attempt to look unconcerned.

'Nothing very bad—eh?'

'Well yes—pretty bad.'

'An—an amputation?'

'No, it's a bigger affair than that.'

'I think—I think they must be expecting me at home.'

'There's no sense funking. If you don't go today you must tomorrow. Better get it over at once. Feel pretty fit?'

'Oh, yes, all right.'

The smile was not a success.

'One more glass of sherry, then. Now come on or we shall be late. I want you to be well in front.'

'Surely that is not necessary.'

'Oh, it is far better. What a drove of students! There are plenty of new men among them. You can tell them easily enough, can't you? If they were going down to be operated upon themselves they could not look whiter.'

'I don't think I should look as white.'

'Well, I was just the same myself. But the feeling soon wears off. You see a fellow with a face like plaster, and before the week is out he is eating his lunch in the dissecting rooms. I'll tell you all about the case when we get to the theatre.'

The students were pouring down the sloping street which led to the infirmary—each with his little sheaf of notebooks in his hand. There were pale, frightened lads, fresh from the High Schools, and callous old chronics, whose generation had passed on and left them. They swept in an unbroken, tumultuous stream from the University gate to the hospital. The figures and gait of the men were young, but there

191

was little youth in most of their faces. Some looked as if they ate too little—a few as if they drank too much. Tall and short, tweed coated and black, round-shouldered, bespectacled and slim, they crowded with clatter of feet and rattle of sticks through the hospital gate. Now and again they thickened into two lines as the carriage of a surgeon of the staff rolled over the cobblestones between.

'There's going to be a crowd at Archer's,' whispered the senior man with suppressed excitement. 'It is grand to see him at work. I've seen him jab all round the aorta until it made me jumpy to watch him. This way, and mind the whitewash.'

They passed under an archway and down a long, stone-flagged corridor with drab coloured doors on either side, each marked with a number. Some of them were ajar, and the novice glanced into them with tingling nerves. He was reassured to catch a glimpse of cheery fires, lines of white-counterpaned beds and a profusion of coloured texts upon the wall. The corridor opened upon a small hall with a fringe of poorly-clad people seated all round upon benches. A young man with a pair of scissors stuck, like a flower, in his button-hole, and a notebook in his hand, was passing from one to the other, whispering and writing.

'Anything good?' asked the third year's man.

'You should have been here yesterday,' said the outpatient clerk, glancing up. 'We had a regular field day. A popliteal aneurysm, a Colles' fracture, a spina bifida, a tropical abscess, and an elephantiasis. How's that for a single haul?'

'I'm sorry I missed it. But they'll come again, I suppose. What's up with the old gentleman?'

A broken workman was sitting in the shadow, rocking himself to and fro and groaning. A woman beside him was trying to console him, patting his shoulder with a hand which was spotted over with curious little white blisters.

'It's a fine carbuncle,' said the clerk, with the air of a connoisseur who describes his orchids to one who can appreciate them. 'It's on his back, and the passage is draughty, so we must not look at it, must we, daddy? Pemphigus,' he added carelessly, pointing to the woman's disfigured hands. 'Would you care to stop and take out a metacarpal?'

'No thank you, we are due at Archer's. Come on;' and they rejoined the throng which was hurrying to the theatre of the famous surgeon.

The tiers of horseshoe benches, rising from the floor to the ceiling, were already packed, and the novice as he entered saw vague, curving lines of faces in front of him, and heard the deep buzz of a hundred voices and sounds of laughter from somewhere up above him. His companion spied an opening on the second bench, and they both squeezed into it.

'This is grand, the senior man whispered; you'll have a rare view of it all.'

Only a single row of heads intervened between them and the operating table. It was of unpainted deal, plain, strong and scrupulously clean. A sheet of brown waterproofing covered half of it, and beneath stood a large tin tray full of sawdust. On the further side, in front of the window, there was a board which was strewed with glittering instruments, forceps, tenacula, saws, canulas and trocars. A line of knives, with long, thin, delicate blades, lay at one side. Two young men lounged in front of this; one threading needles, the other doing something to a brass coffee-pot-like thing which hissed out puffs of steam.

'That's Peterson,' whispered the senior. 'The big, bald man in the front row. He's the skin-grafting man, you know. And that's Anthony Browne, who took a larynx out successfully last winter. And there's Murphy the pathologist, and Stoddart the eye man. You'll come to know them all soon.'

'Who are the two men at the table?'

'Nobody—dressers. One has charge of the instruments and the other of the puffing billy. It's Lister's antiseptic spray, you know, and Archer's one of the carbolic acid men. Hayes is the leader of the cleanliness-and-cold-water school, and they all hate each other like poison.'

A flutter of interest passed through the closely-packed benches as a woman in petticoat and bodice was led in by two nurses. A red wollen shawl was draped over her head and round her neck. The face which looked out from it was that of a woman in the prime of her years, but drawn with suffering and of peculiar bees-wax tint. Her head drooped as she walked, and one of the nurses, with her arm round her waist, was whispering consolation in her ear. She gave a quick side glance at the instrument table as she passed, but the nurses turned her away from it.

'What ails her? asked the novice.'

'Cancer of the parotid. It's the devil of a case, extends right away back behind the carotids. There's hardly a man but Archer would dare follow it. Ah, here he is himself.'

As he spoke, a small brisk, iron-grey man came striding into the room, rubbing his hands together as he walked. He had a clean-shaven face of the naval officer type, with large, bright eyes, and a firm, straight mouth. Behind him came his big house surgeon with his gleaming pince-nez and a trail of dressers, who grouped themselves into the corners of the room.

'Gentleman,' cried the surgeon in a voice as hard and brisk as his manner. 'We have here an interesting case of tumour of the parotid, originally cartilaginous but now assuming malignant characteristics, and therefore requiring excision. On to the table, nurse! Thank you! Chloroform, clerk! Thank you! You can take the shawl off, nurse.'

The woman lay back upon the waterproofed pillow and her murderous tumour lay revealed. In itself it was a pretty thing, ivory white with a mesh of blue veins, and curving gently from jaw to chest. But the lean, yellow face, and the stringy throat were in horrible contrast with the plumpness and sleekness of this monstrous growth. The surgeon placed a hand on each side of it and pressed it slowly backwards and forwards.

'Adherent at one place, gentlemen,' he cried. 'The growth involves the carotids and jugulars, and passes behind the ramus of the jaw, whither we must be prepared to follow it. It is impossible to say how deep our dissection may carry us. Carbolic tray, thank you! Dressings of carbolic gauze, if you please! Push the chloroform, Mr Johnson. Have the small saw ready in case it is necessary to remove the jaw.'

The patient was moaning gently under the towel which had been placed over her face. She tried to raise her arms and to draw up her knees but two dressers restrained her. The heavy air was full of the penetrating smells of carbolic acid and of chloroform. A muffled cry came from under the towel and then a snatch of a song, sung in a high, quavering, monotonous voice.

He say, says he,
If you fly with me
 You'll be the mistress of the ice-cream van;
 You'll be the mistress of the—

It mumbled off into a drone and stopped. The surgeon came across, still rubbing his hands, and spoke to an elderly man in front of the novice.

'Narrow squeak for the Government,' he said.

'Oh, ten is enough.'

'They won't have ten long. They'd do better to resign before they are driven to it.'

'Oh, I should fight it out.'

'What's the use. They can't get past the committee, even if they get a vote in the House. I was talking to—'

'Patient's ready, sir, said the dresser.'

'Talking to M'Donald—but I'll tell you about it presently.'

He walked back to the patient, who was breathing in long, heavy gasps. 'I propose,' said he, passing his hand over the tumour in an almost caressing fashion, 'to make a free incision over the posterior border and to take another forward at right angles to the lower end of it. Might I trouble you for a medium knife, Mr. Johnson.'

The novice, with eyes which were dilating with horror saw the surgeon pick up the long, gleaming knife, dip it into a tin basin and balance it in his fingers as an artist might his brush. Then he saw him pinch up the skin above the tumour with his left hand. At the sight, his nerves, which had already been tried once or twice that day, gave way utterly. His head swam round and he felt that in another instant he might faint. He dared not look at the patient. He dug his thumbs into his ears less some scream should come to haunt him, and he fixed his eyes rigidly upon the wooden ledge in front of him. One glance, one cry, would, he knew, break down the shred of self-possession which he still retained. He tried to think of cricket, of green fields and rippling water, of his sisters at home— of anything rather than of what was going on so near him.

And yet, somehow, even with his ears stopped up, sounds seemed to penetrate to him and to carry their own tale. He heard, or thought he heard, the long hissing of the carbolic engine. Then he was conscious of some movement among the dressers. Were there groans too breaking in upon him, and some other sound, some fluid sound which was more dreadfully suggestive still? His mind would keep building up every step of the operation, and fancy made it more ghastly than fact could have been. His nerves tingled and quivered. Minute by minute the giddiness grew more marked, the numb, sickly feeling at his heart more distressing. And then suddenly, with a groan, his head pitching forward and his brow cracking sharply upon the narrow, wooden shelf in front of him, he lay in a dead faint.

When he came to himself he was lying in the empty theatre with his collar and shirt undone. The third year's man was dabbing a wet sponge over his face, and a couple of grinning dressers were looking on.

'All right,' cried the novice, sitting up and rubbing his eyes; 'I'm sorry to have made an ass of myself.'

'Well, so I should think,' said his companion. 'What on earth did you faint about?'

'I couldn't help it. It was that operation.'

'What operation?'

'Why, that cancer.'

There was a pause, and then the three students burst out laughing.

'Why, you juggins,' cried the senior man, 'there never was an operation at all. They found the patient didn't stand the chloroform well, and so the whole thing was off. Archer has been giving us one of his racy lectures, and you fainted just in the middle of his favourite story.'

REFERENCES
Goldman M 1987 *Lister Ward* (Bristol: Adam Hilger) pp 70–7

Conan Doyle A 1934 *Round the Red Lamp* 2nd edn (London) pp 9–19
Conan Doyle A 1930 *Memories and Adventures* 2nd edn (London) p. 33

Mr Chamberlen's Secret

It was not very ethical, for an English accoucheur as famous as Hugh I Chamberlen, momentarily in Paris, to try and sell to the French Government (for 10 000 *scudi*) a family secret jealously held for nearly a century. It was, he argued, a portentous secret: an instrument with which a woman in labour 'could be delivered in eight minutes'. Hugh's motivation for effecting the sale was anything but humanitarian. His whole family was heavily involved in the consequences of a financial disaster amounting to bankruptcy. At the time (1670), obstetrical and perinatal mortality were rampant in Paris; and the Government, well aware of the fact, was more concerned with actuarial figures than with Dr Chamberlen's questionable ethics. Thus a meeting was arranged between the owner of the secret instrument and Dr F Mauriceau, then regarded as 'the oracle of accoucheurs of his century'. And who can tell that it was not Mauriceau himself, aware of Chamberlen's practices, to attract him to France—partly to find out more about the business and partly, perhaps, to discredit him with malice aforethought?

Right then, the French accoucheur had been called upon to assist a woman in childbirth: a primiparous dwarf with a pelvis so narrow and misshapen as to make vaginal delivery practically impossible. Hence the agreement: should Dr Chamberlen succeed in delivering the dwarf with his secret instrument, Mauriceau would authorise payment of the sum requested; otherwise, the instrument would be forever condemned.

So on 19 August 1670 an apparently confident Dr Chamberlen shut himself in a room with the poor dwarf in labour. But after three hours of torturing as well as fruitless attempts at extracting the fetus (by then mercifully dead) with his forceps, he was forced to admit defeat; and clinical disaster was compounded soon afterwards, when a Caesarean section was made and the mother also died.

CHAMBERLEN ENTERPRISE

Chamberlen was not a complete stranger to France. His great-grandparents were in fact French. Probably the whole blame for what follows must be fixed on a wooden splinter from a spear, which penetrated the visor of King Henry the Second of France during a tournament and gouged out one of his eyes—in consequence of which the sovereign died. The ill-fated monarch was succeeded by François II, a sickly teenager who promised a world of religious tolerance but soon fell to persecuting the Protestants (called Huguenots after the corrupted German *eidgnoss*, or 'confederate'), a party that was active in Geneva in the XVI century.

There were three wars against the Huguenots in France between 1562 and 1570. At last in 1572 Catherine de Medici (then regent for her second-born son Charles IX, after the sudden death of the first-born Francis II), organised an attempt on the life of Admiral Gaspard de Coligny, chief of the Huguenots; but the killer failed, merely wounding his victim. Obviously the Huguenots made a great ado about this, with loud demands that those responsible be punished. Things like that are bound to end badly. Catherine ordered a massacre. And sure enough, on the feast of St Bartholomew (24 August 1572) 3000 Huguenots were butchered in Paris and 15 000 more in the provinces. Many survivors, smelling trouble, left France in a hurry. Some migrated to North America (where they colonised North and South Carolina); others scattered throughout Europe. Some, more enlightened than others, had left France before the massacre—among them the surgeon and accoucheur William Chamberlen, who fled Paris with his wife Geneviève and son Peter I in 1569 to repair first to Southampton, later to London.

It seems that the original family name was Chambrelein—at least, it is so spelled in the actuary books of the French Church at Southampton; later documents show the name variously as Chambellan, Chamberlain, or Chamberleine. William's sons always signed their name 'Chamberlan'; the great-grandchildren switched to 'Chamberlen'. The family founder's name must have been Villame Chambrelein. After fleeing France, he had two more children, one again named Peter and so becoming Peter II.

It was probably Peter I who constructed with his own hands the instrument from which the obstetric forceps was derived: a 'noble tool capable of limiting human suffering and saving more lives than any other in the surgical armamentarium'. The instrument made by Peter I consisted simply of two curved iron blades shaped somewhat like two spoons. Simple as it was, the tool was guarded as a family secret for fully three generations, or almost one century. When Peter I or one of his obstetrical epigones went abroad to deliver a woman in labour, they did not carry the forceps in their bag. No sir: they had it carried by two strong men in an apparently heavy wooden chest ornamented with gold inlays, or transported on a special coach to increase mystery and make people talk. What Peter's original instrument looked like was discovered by mere chance in 1813, a century and a half after his death, when a hidden trap-door was found in his old house at Woodham Mortimer Hall, Essex County, leading to a hollow space between the floor and the ceiling below. And there was a large box full of odds and ends: old letters, trinkets, coins, fans—and as you have guessed, no fewer than four pairs of obstetrical forceps. One was just a rough-hewn model, possibly an experimental prototype. The other three consisted of two flat metal levers curved to fit the fetal head. The two levers could be placed separately into the birth canal and then hinged together for better purchase and more effective pulling. Perhaps the main intuition of Peter I was to exploit the fact that once the fetal head was extracted, the rest would follow without any difficulty.

That the secrets of forceps handling be divulged by indiscreet observers was practically impossible since no outsiders were ever admitted to the delivery room and the woman herself was carefully blindfolded. So Peter I became rich and famous and had many illustrious customers, including Queen Anne and Mary Henrietta, wife of Charles I of England.

Peter II was second to none. He was admitted with his elder brother to the Barber Surgeon's Company of London, where the two were noted not only because of their professional abilities but also because of their quarrelsome and greedy disposition. Their proposal of creating an association of London midwives was rejected by the College of Physicians on the grounds that it was motivated by personal interest, namely trying to monopolise the profession for the sake of gain. The College also mentioned a 'deprecable family secret' that was handed on from father to son ('. . . *It seems they use metal instruments* . . .'). Neither brother abode by the laws of regulatory agencies. In 1612 Peter I was prosecuted by the Barber Surgeon's Company for illicit practice of the medical profession and jailed at Newgate, later freed by intercession of the Queen and Archbishop of Canterbury; and Peter II was investigated for the same reason in 1620.

MIDWIVES INCORPORATED

Another example of Chamberlen enterprise was the son of Peter II, named Peter III (the Chamberlens seemed to lack imagination in naming their offspring—they called almost everybody Peter and gave each Peter a consecutive number). Peter III (soon nicknamed 'Doctor Peter') started his medical studies at age 14 at the Emmanuel College of Cambridge and continued them at Heidelberg and Padua, where he obtained his doctorate in 1619. In 1628 he was admitted to the Royal College of Physicians—upon condition that he change his 'eccentric way of dressing' and adopt the sober garb of his fellow-members. In 1630 he succeeded his uncle as Royal Accoucheur, later to manage the birth of King Charles II.

Doctor Peter, however, was also famous for another enterprise. Revamping the old idea of Daddy and Uncle, he approached London midwives with promises of benefits galore if they would make a Corporation where he himself would train them and give them a patent. In return, the ineffable Master would graciously accept a tax or levy on each delivery conducted by one of his certified pupils; and of course he would be summoned to attend all difficult deliveries. The idea was not entirely without merit. The need was felt throughout Europe for some sort of training and qualification of *commères*, for centuries a breed of practical 'old hands' completely innocent of medical knowledge. It seems that the first 'sworn' or certified midwife was Madame Louise Bourgeois, the wife of a French surgeon, who in the latter part of the XVI century asked permission to attend the *Hôtel Dieu* for five years; after which she was examined by a committee of physicians who made her a 'sworn and patented *accoucheuse*', or certified midwife. (At the time, ignorant 'collecting midwives' were heard in court as 'expert witnesses'.) Madame Bourgeois' training enabled her to assist Catherine de Medici when she gave birth to the future Louis XIII, write articles on obstetrics (she gave a good description of face presentation) and discuss head conversion—to which she preferred podalic version.

In Italy Scipione Mercuri devoted himself to obstetrics. Being a man of the cloth, he was strongly opposed by his brethren, who could hardly tolerate that a minister of God should busy himself with the female genital function. Scipione, however, worked steadily toward making the obstetrician's position official—lest, perhaps, he should suffer the fate of Hamburg's Dr Wertt, who had been burned alive in 1552 for assisting, disguised in feminine garb, a woman in labour—woe to the man who would dare so much in those times!

HUGH I SELLS HIS SECRET

In England, also, things were slowly turning to the advantage of people like the Chamberlens. Peter II (who lived to be 82) had three sons: Hugh I, Paul and John. And Hugh I (the future father of Hugh II) began to meditate that he could live like a prince if he succeeded in selling the family secret: hence his trip to Paris and trial by ordeal on Mauriceau's poor dwarf woman. The fiasco was nothing short of grandiose. But Hugh I was not a man to be easily discouraged. He hooked up a Dutch obstetrician, Eric van Roonhuyze, and gave him a swindle most memorable, as we shall see in a moment.

199

His professional background, as you will have guessed, was far from adamantine. He had his own queer theories about treating diseases—at one point the Royal College of Physicians enjoined that he submit to board examinations for authority to practice medicine; but he ignored the summons. Later on, he was inquired over the death of a woman with pneumonia, whom he had 'treated' by bloodletting, diaphoretics, purgatives, and emetics. Then he was removed from the post of Royal Accoucheur on the grounds that when the Queen gave birth to James III, he was late in arriving at Court!

Now about the swindle. Some 50 years after the sale of his 'secret' to van Roonhuyze, the latter resold it to two well-meaning physicians, de Visscher and van de Poll, who intended to divulge it. And after disbursing the handsome sum requested, they found themselves holding nothing more than a plain metal lever. So it became apparent that, in order to preserve his superiority on all other obstetricians, Hugh I had not even sold his forceps to van Roonhuyze, but only a piece of iron!

Be that as it may, Hugh I should be credited with being the first to make public mention of his family secret:

> My father, my brothers and myself (but no one else in Europe) have by the grace of God and our own industry developed an instrument which we have been using for a long time to deliver women in childbirth, in cases of head presentation, without any risk to them or the infants; whereas others must place in jeopardy, if not destroy with hooks, one or the other life, or both.

So started the great adventure of the obstetrical forceps. Rogier van Roonhuyze (the son of the original buyer), himself an obstetrician, had a good flair for business. For a suitable consideration he would sell his secret to a few close friends, who would in turn resell it to others. The traffic became so important that it came to involve the Amsterdam College of Physicians and Pharmacists, in the form of a 1746 decree to the effect that no one could deliver children who could not demonstrate that he was in possession of 'the secret'—which the examiners themselves were currently selling for 2000–2500 guldens a throw!

REFERENCE

Sterpellone L 1986 *Instruments for Health* (Farmitalia Carlo Erba: Freiburg i. Br.) pp 28–36

First Orbiting Space Mausoleum Okayed

The US government yesterday approved an American consortium's plan to rocket the cremated remains of 10330 people into space for a fee of $3900 each.

The Transportation Department announced tentative approval for a commercially built rocket launch of the world's first space mausoleum from Wallops Island, Virginia, by mid-1987.

'It doesn't interfere with national defence, with international treaty obligations or with public health and safety,' a Transportation Department spokeswoman said.

While plans for the unique venture have been approved, she said, ashes of those who want to circle the earth or rest among the stars will not be launched until final technical details are reviewed.

REFERENCE
The *Bangkok World* 13 February 1985

Man Become Violent After Eating Crisps

An allergy to potatoes caused a 'pleasant and likeable' young Irishman to change into a 'surly and aggressive individual,' a court heard yesterday.

Tony Doherty, 24, was charged in March with assaulting his father whom he tried to strangle with a tie after eating two packets of crisps, Belfast Crown Court was told.

Doherty, of Ballymacombs Road, Portglenone, Co. Antrim, admitted the offence but sentence was deferred because of suspicion about an allergy.

Imposing a two-year conditional discharge on Doherty, Judge Peter Gibson called the case 'a highly exceptional one.'

REFERENCE
The *Daily Telegraph* 20 September 1986

Anatomical Rhyming Slang

Rhyming slang is not only limited to London's Cockney population, but is also used in Australia and in the American underworld, and occasionally in Ireland. When spoken, the second word of the two-word phrase is omitted and therefore sounds like some sort of unintelligible code to those new to rhyming slang.

In some cases there are more than one or two rhyming phrases for the same part of the anatomy. Thus for *leg* there are *clothes* peg, *Scotch* peg, *Dutch* peg, *bacon* and egg, *fried* egg; and for the famous four-letter word there are *friar* tuck, *colonial* puck, *goose* and duck. Parts of London are sometimes used as in *Hounslow* Heath or *Hampstead* Heath for *teeth*; *Barnet* Fair for hair; and *Hampton* Wick for *penis* or alternatively *almond* rock or *giggle* stick. The origin is not always clear and for *goose* and duck, Franklyn in his *Dictionary of Rhyming Slang* gives the following logical reasoning! The term was current in 1944 on the Pacific Coast of America but it is assumed by Americans to be of English origin. It is not now used in London and there is never any trace of it having been. It is emphatically not known in Australia. Therefore, it must be Irish.

Hair = Barnet Fair
Head = alive or dead
Ear = Melbourne pier, bottle of beer, sighs and tears
Eyes = mince pies
Face = boat race
Nose = ruby rose, these and those
Tongue = heart and lung, brewers bung
Forehead = centre lead
Lips = apple pips
Mouth = north and south
Teeth = Hounslow Heath, Hampstead Heath
Chin = Gunga Din
Neck = bushel and peck
Throat = hairy goat
Moustache = dot and dash
Hand = German band
Breast = Bristol City
Feet = plates of meat
Knees = bugs and fleas
Testicles = cobblers awls, cobblers stalls
Penis = almond rock, giggle stick, Hampton Wick
Leg = clothes peg, Scotch peg, Dutch peg, bacon and egg, fried egg
Anus = Khyber Pass, Elephant and Castle

A few medical conditions are also the subject for rhyming slang such as:

Syphilis (pox) = coachman on the box
Gonorrhoea (clap) = hat and cap
Deaf = Mutt and Jeff
Gout = salmon and trout, in and out

REFERENCE
Franklyn J 1975 *A Dictionary of Rhyming Slang* (London: Routledge and
    Kegan Paul)

The Death of John Partridge in 1708

A London man called John Partridge, who claimed to be an
astrologer, was publishing predictions in the form of almanacs, which
prognostications annoyed Dean Swift because they were, he felt,

simply Whig political propaganda. Accordingly, in 1708, Swift produced a rival almanac in which he forecast the death of Partridge on 29 March. Then on 30 March he published an eyewitness account of Partridge's death together with a funeral elegy. Partridge indignantly protested and advertised in the papers that he was still alive. Swift retorted in a *vindication* proving that the poor man was really dead, and other writers took up the cry. In the end, no one believed the unhappy Partridge, and so, in effect, he ceased to exist.

Anecdote of The Earl of Shrewsbury and a Mouse

John Talbot, Earl of Shrewsbury, born near Whitchurch in 1373, was a renowned soldier who, after many battles, fell at Castillon at the battle of Bordeaux in 1453. Shakespeare in *Henry VI*, Act 2, describes him as:

> The scourge of France,
> The Talbot so much feared abroad,
> That with his name, the mothers still their babes.

Even after his death, the old soldier has remained the focus of much interest and controversy. He was buried initially at Rouen and 50 years later his heart, which was embalmed separately, and his bones were brought to Whitchurch and buried in the church, with his heart lying under the porch.

In 1874 his tomb was restored and at a solemn ceremony the bones were reinterred. Great interest was aroused at the condition of the old warrior's remains, for he was discovered to be resting not in a coffin, but in a strong box three feet long, which soon crumbled to dust on exposure to air. It was found that every bone, from the skull to the smallest metacarpal, had carefully been wrapped in rare cloth, and in the skull itself was found the body of a mummified mouse with her three young ones.

An interesting controversy ensued. A prominent dental surgeon insisted that it must have been a French Catholic mouse which had found its way through the base of the skull before the bones had been prepared for burial. The then Rector of St Alkmund's Church disagreed, and claimed to have found torn leaves of an English Prayer Book in the mouse's nest and a gnawed hole in the cloth on which the skull was wrapped. The fatal gash in the Earl's skull provided the access point. It was an Anglican mouse! Whatever the religion, though, the mummified mouse was awarded an inscription:

A mighty mountain from its womb one day,
With groanings loud brought forth a mouse they say:
The skull which once upreared great Talbot's crest
Gashed by a foeman, gave this mouse a nest.

REFERENCE
Adapted from *A Short History and Guide of the Parish Church of St. Alkmund, Whitchurch, Shropshihre* 1978

Florence Nightingale and the Crimean War Hospitals, 1854–6

Miss Nightingale reported the arrival of her expedition at Constantinople in a short note to her parents:—

Constantinople, *November* 4, on board *Vectis.*—Dearest People—Anchored off the Seraglio point, waiting for our fate whether we can disembark direct into the Hospital, which, with our heterogeneous mass, we should prefer.

At six o'clock yesterday morn I staggered on deck to look at the plains of Troy, the tomb of Achilles, the mouths of the Scamander, the little harbour of Tenedos, between which and the mainshore our *Vectis*, with steward's cabins and galley torn away, blustering, creaking, shrieking, storming, rushed on her way. It was in a dense mist that the ghosts of the Trojans answered my cordial hail, through which the old Gods, nevertheless, peered down from the hill of Ida upon their old plain. My enthusiasm for the heroes though was undiminished by wind and wave.

We made the castles of Europe and Asia (Dardanelles) by eleven, but also reached Constantinople this morn in a thick and heavy rain, through which the Sophia, Sulieman, the Seven Towers, the walls, and the Golden Horn looked like a bad daguerrotype washed out.

We have not yet heard what the Embassy or Military Hospital have done for us, nor received our orders.

Bad news from Balaclava. You will hear the awful wreck of our poor cavalry, 400 wounded, arriving *at this moment* for us to nurse. We have just built another hospital at the Dardanelles.

You will want to know about our crew. One has turned out ill, others will do.

(*Later*) Just starting for Scutari. We are to be housed in the Hospital this very afternoon. Everybody is most kind. The fresh wounded are, I believe, to be placed under our care. They are landing them now.

The Hospital, to which Miss Nightingale refers, was to be the chief scene of her labours for the next six months, and a few particulars about it and other hospitals, in which the nursing was under her superintendence, must be given in order to make future proceedings intelligible. The principal hospitals of the British army during the Crimean War—four in number—were at Scutari (or in its immediate neighbourhood), the suburb of mournful beauty which looks across to Constantinople from the Asiatic side of the Bosphorus.

The first hospital to be established was in the Turkish Military Hospital. This was made over to the British in May 1854, and was called by them *The General Hospital*. Having been originally designed for a hospital, and being given up to the English partially fitted, it was, wrote Miss Nightingale, 'reduced to good order early, by the unwearied efforts of the first-class Staff Surgeon in introducing a good working system. It was then maintained in excellent condition till the close of the war.' It had accommodation for 1000 patients, but the Battle of the Alma showed that much larger accommodation would be wanted.

North of the General Hospital, and near to the famous Turkish cemetery of Scutari, are the Selimiyeh Barracks—a great yellow building with square towers at each angle. This building was made over to the British for use as a hospital after the Battle of the Alma, and by them was always called *The Barrack Hospital*. This is the hospital in which Miss Nightingale and her band of female nurses were first established, and in which she herself had her headquarters throughout her stay at Scutari. It is built on rising ground, in a beautiful situation, looking over the Sea of Marmora on one side, towards the Princes' Islands on another, and towards Constantinople and up the Bosphorus on a third. 'I have not been out of the Hospital Walls yet,' wrote Miss Nightingale ten days after her arrival, 'but the most beautiful view in all the world, I believe, lies outside.' Her quarters were in the north-west tower, on the left of the Main Guard (or principal entrance). There was a large kitchen or storeroom, of which we shall hear more presently, and out of it on either side various other rooms opened. Mr Bracebridge and the courier slept in one small room; Miss Nightingale and Mrs Bracebridge in another. The nurses slept in other rooms. The whole space occupied by Miss Nightingale and her nurses was about equal to that allotted to three medical officers and their servants, or to that occupied by the Commandant. 'This was done,' she explained, 'in order to make no pressure for room on an already overcrowded hospital. It could not have been done with justice to the women's health, had not Miss Nightingale later taken a house in Scutari at private expense, to which every nurse attacked with fever was removed.' The quarters were as uncomfortable as they were cramped. 'Occasionally,' wrote Miss

Nightingale, 'our roof is torn off, or the windows are blown in, and we are under water for the night.' The Hospital was infested also with rodents and vermin; and, among other new accomplishments acquired under the stress of new occasions, Miss Nightingale became an expert rat-killer. This skill was afterwards called into use at Balaclava. In the spring of 1856, one of the nuns whom she had taken with her to the Crimea—Sister Mary Martha—had a dangerous attack of fever. Miss Nightingale nursed the case; and one night, while watching by the sick-bed, she saw a large rat upon the rafters over the Sister's head; she succeeded in knocking it down and killing it, without disturbing the patient. The condition of physical discomfort in which, surrounded by terrible scenes of suffering, she had to do her work, should be remembered in taking the measure of her fortitude and devotion.

The maximum number of patients accommodated at any one time (Dec. 23, 1854) in the Barrack Hospital was 2434. It was half-an-hour's walk from the General Hospital, and an invalided soldier records that he used to accompany Miss Nightingale from one hospital to another in order to light her home on wet stormy nights, across the barren common which lay between them.

Farther south of the General Hospital, in the quarter of Haidar Pasha, was what was known as *The Palace Hospital*, consisting of various buildings belonging to the Sultan's Summer Palace. These were occupied as a hospital in January 1855. Miss Nightingale had no responsibility here; but in the summer of 1855, the female nursing of sick officers, quartered in one of these buildings, was placed under the superintendence of Mrs Willoughby Moore, the widow of an officer who had died a noble death in the war, and four female nurses, sent out specially from England.

Finally, there were hospitals at *Koulali*, four or five miles farther north, upon the same Asiatic shore of the Bosphorus. These hospitals were opened in December 1854. The nursing in them was originally under Miss Nightingale's supervision, but she was presently relieved of it. The hospitals were broken up in November 1855, when, of the female nursing establishment, a portion went home, and the rest passed under Miss Nightingale into the hospitals at Scutari.

There were also five hospitals in the Crimea, but particulars of these may be deferred till the time comes for following Miss Nightingale upon her expeditions to the front. For the nursing in the Civil Military Hospitals at Renkioi (on the Dardanelles) and at Smyrna, and for the Naval Hospital at Therapia, Miss Nightingale had no responsibility, though there is voluminous correspondence among her papers showing that she was constantly consulted upon the site and arrangements of these hospitals. The medical superintendent of the hospital at Renkioi was Dr E A Parkes, with whom Miss Nightingale formed a friendship which endured to the end of his life.

The state of the hospitals when Miss Nightingale arrived requires some description, which, however, need not be long. The treatment of the sick and wounded during the Crimean War was the subject of Departmental Inquiries, Select Committees, and Royal Commissions, which, when they had finished sitting upon the hospitals, began sitting upon each other. Enormous piles of Blue-books were accumulated, and in the course of my work I have disturbed much dust upon them. The conduct of every department and every individual concerned was the subject of charge, answer, and countercharge innumerable. Each generation deserves, no doubt, the records of mal-administration which it gets; but one generation need not be punished by having to examine in detail the records of another. Some of the details of the Crimean muddle will indeed necessarily be disinterred in the course of our story; but all that need here be collected from the heaps aforesaid are three general conclusions.

The reader must remember, in the first place, that, apart from controverted particulars, it was made abundantly manifest that there was gross neglect in the service of the sick and wounded. The conflict of testimony is readily intelligible. It was easy to give an account based upon the facts of one hospital or of one time which was not applicable to another. At Scutari, for instance, the General Hospital was from the first better ordered than the Barrack Hospital. Then, again, different witnesses had different standards of what was 'good' in War Hospitals; to some, anything was good if it was no worse than the standard of the Peninsular War. Of Sir George Brown, who commanded the Light Division in the Crimea, it was said: 'As he was thrown into a cart on some straw when shot through the legs in Spain, he thinks the same conveyances admirable now, and hates ambulances as the invention of the Evil One.' Miss Nightingale had much indignant sarcasm for those who seemed content that the soldier in hospital should be placed in the condition of 'former wars,' instead of perceiving that he 'should be treated with that degree of decency and humanity which the improved feeling of the nineteenth century demands.' But the principal reason for the conflict of testimony was that the very facts of protest and inquiry put all the officials concerned upon the defensive. Any suggestion of default or defect was resented as a personal imputation. There is a curious illustration in the letter which the Head of the Army Medical Department wrote to his Principal Medical Officer in view of the Roebuck Committee. 'I beg you to supply me, and that immediately'—with what? with the truth, the whole truth, and nothing but the truth? No—'with every kind of information which you may deem likely to enable me to establish a character for it [the Department], which the public appear desirous to prove that it does not possess.' But though there was much conflict of evidence, the final verdict was decisive. What Greville wrote in his Journal—'the accounts published in the *Times* turn out to be true'—was established by official inquiry and admitted by Ministers. In consequence of the indictment in the *Times*, a Commission of Inquiry was dispatched to the East by the Secretary of State. The Commission arrived at Constantinople simultaneously with Miss Nightingale, and four months later it reported to the Duke of Newcastle. I need not trouble here with many particulars of its Report; for they were adopted and confirmed by a Select Committee of the House of Commons a few months later (the famous 'Roebuck Committee'), which pronounced succinct sentence that 'the state of the hospitals was disgraceful.' The ships which brought the sick and wounded from the Crimea were painfully ill-equipped. The voyage from Balaclava to Scutari usually took eight days and a half. During the first four months of the war, there died on a voyage, no longer than from Tynemouth to London, 74 out of every 1000 embarked. The landing arrangements added to the men's sufferings. To an unpractised eye the buildings used as hospitals at Scutari were imposing and convenient; and this fact accounts for some of the rose-coloured descriptions by which persons in high places were for a time misled. Even the Principal Medical Officer on the spot was naively content with whitewash as a preparation to fit the Barrack for use as a hospital. In fact, however,

One of the wards in the hospital at Scutari, from a coloured lithograph by Simpson. (Courtesy Mansell Collection.)

the buildings were pest-houses. Underneath the great structures 'were sewers of the worst possible construction, loaded with filth, mere cesspools, in fact, through which the wind blew sewer air up the pipes of numerous open privies into the corridors and wards where the sick were lying.' There was also frightful overcrowding. For many months the space for each patient was one-fourth of what it ought to have been. And there was no proper ventilation. 'It is impossible,' Miss Nightingale told the Royal Commission of 1857, 'to describe the state of the atmosphere of the Barrack Hospital at night. I have been well acquainted with the dwellings of the worst parts of most of the great cities in Europe, but have never been in any atmosphere which I could compare with it.' Lastly, hospital comforts, and even many hospitals necessaries, were deficient. The supply of bedsteads was inadequate. The commonest utensils, for decency as well as for comfort, were lacking. The sheets, said Miss Nightingale, 'were of canvas, and so coarse that the wounded men begged to be left in their blankets. It was indeed impossible to put men in such a state of emaciation into those sheets. There was no bedroom furniture of any kind, and only empty beer or wine bottles for candle-sticks.' Necessary surgical and medical appliances were often either wanting or not forthcoming. There was no machinery, until Miss Nightingale came, for providing any hospital delicacies. The result of this state of things upon patients arriving after a painful voyage in an extreme state of weakness and emaciation, from wounds, from frost-bite, from dysentery, may be imagined, and it is no wonder that cholera and typhus were rife. In February 1855 the mortality per cent of the cases treated was forty-two. No words are necessary to emphasize so terrible a figure.

Mr Herbert had not waited for the reports of Commission and Committee to reach the conclusion that things were wrong:—

'I have for some time,' he wrote on December 14, 1854, to the Commandant at Scutari, 'been very anxious and very much dissatisfied as to the state of the hospital. I believe that every effort has been made by the medical men, and I hear that you have been indefatigable in the conduct of the immediate business of your department. But there has been evidently a want of co-operation between departments, and a fear of responsibility or timidity, arising from an entire misconception of the wishes of the Government. No expense has been spared at home, and immense stores are sent out, but they are not forthcoming. Some are at Varna, and for some inexplicable reason they are not brought down to Scutari. When stores are in the hospital, they are not issued without forms so cumbrous as to make the issue unavailing through delay. The Purveyor's staff is said to be insufficient. The Commissariat staff is said to be insufficient, your own staff is said to be insufficient,' etc.

By admission, then, and by official sentence, there were things amiss

210

at Scutari which urgently called for amendment. This is the first general conclusion which has to be remembered in relation to Miss Nightingale's work.

To what individuals the disgrace of 'a disgraceful state of things' attached, it is happily no concern of ours here to inquire. But as I have called Mr Sidney Herbert as a witness to the fact of the disgrace, I must add my conviction that his own part in the business was wholly beneficent. Some research among the documents entitles me, perhaps, to express entire agreement with Mr Kinglake's remark upon 'what might have been if the Government, instead of appointing a Commission of *enquiry* on the 23rd of October, had then delegated Mr Sidney Herbert to go out for a month to the Bosphorus, and there *dictate* immediate action.' At home, Mr Herbert was a good man struggling in the toils. The fact is that, though there were some individuals palpably to blame, the real fault was everybody's or nobody's. It was the fault of a vicious system, or rather the vice was that there was no system at all, no co-ordination, but only division of responsibility. The remarks of Mr Herbert, just quoted, point to the evil, and on every page of the Blue-books it is written large. There were at least eight authorities, working independently of each other, whose co-operation was yet necessary to get anything well done. There was the Secretary of State; there was the War Office; there were the Horse Guards, the Ordnance, the Victualling Office, the Transport Office, the Army Medical Department, and the Treasury. The Director-General of the Medical Department in London told the Roebuck Committee that he was under five distinct masters—the Commander-in-Chief, the Secretary of State, the Secretary-at-War, the Master-General of Ordnance, and the Board of Ordnance. The Secretary of State said that he had issued no instructions as to the hospitals; he had left that to the Medical Board. But the Medical Director-General said that it would have been impertinent for him to take the first step. If I were writing the history of the Crimean War, or of the Government Offices, other fundamental reasons for the disgraceful state of things in the hospitals—notably the miscalculated plan of military campaign—would have to be taken into account; but I am writing only the life of Miss Nightingale, and all that under this head the reader need be asked to bear in mind is this: That the root of the evils which had to be dealt with was division of responsibility, and reluctance to assume it.

The third conclusion of the official inquiries, which I want to emphasize, is contained in a passage in the Roebuck Committee's Report, which prefaced a reference to Miss Nightingale's mission: 'Your Committee in conclusion cannot but remark that the first real improvements in the lamentable condition of the hospitals at Scutari are to be attributed to private suggestions, private exertions, and private benevolence.'

So, then, we see that there were disgraceful evils at Scutari needing amendment, and that in order to amend them what was needed was bold initiative. This it was that Miss Nightingale supplied. The popular voice thought of her only or mainly as the gentle nurse. That, too, she was; and to her self-devotion in applying a woman's insight to a new sphere, a portion of her fame must ever be ascribed. But when men who knew all the facts spoke of her 'commanding genius,' it was rather of her work as an administrator that they were thinking. 'They could scarcely realize without personally seeing it,' Mr Stafford told the House of Commons, 'the heartfelt gratitude of the soldiers, or the amount of misery which had been relieved' by Miss Nightingale and her nurses; and, he added, 'it was impossible to do justice, not only to the kindness of heart, but to the clever judgment, the ready intelligence, and the experience displayed by the distinguished lady to whom this difficult mission had been entrusted.' These were the qualities which enabled her to reform, or to be the inspirer and instigator of reforms in, the British system of military hospitals. She began her work, where it lay immediately to her hand, in the Barrack Hospital at Scutari. She did the work in three ways. She applied an expert's touch and a woman's insight to a hospital hitherto managed exclusively by men. She boldly assumed responsibility, and did things herself which she could find no one else ready to do. And, thirdly, she was instant and persistent in suggestion, exhortation, reproaches, addressed to the authorities at home.

REFERENCE
Cook E 1913 *The Life of Florence Nightingale* vol. I (1820–1861) (London: Macmillan) pp 171–81

A Dropped Catch—The Case of the Bouncing Baby

The second child I ever delivered slipped between my trembling fingers and fell head first into the bucket. To this day, those gleaming steel receptacles stationed three feet below the bulging perineum remind me of that awesome moment in 1959. The noise of impact of head against bucket has remained with me throughout my obstetrical career.

Of all the sensory stimuli, a noise is the most difficult to describe in writing. If you are prepared to drop a large turnip into a pail containing one inch (2.5 cm) of water, you will get some idea of the sound the baby's head produced. The metallic plop was followed by a momentary silence lasting a thousand years. There was an anguished cry from the widwife. No one, in living memory, had dropped a babe before. Neonatal baby battering by budding obstetricians had not, as yet, been recorded in the literature.

'Call the house surgeon! Fetch the paediatric house officer! Tell the midwifery sister I want her immediately!' The demands were rattled out with sten-gun precision. 'And you, Mr McGarry, pick up that infant and place it on the cot before the mother stops breathing the gas and air.'

This I did; the infant was by now crying lustily and, with hindsight, I admit that the cry had a hurtful note about it—rather like a four-year-old who has dropped his ice-cream down a roadside drain.

'Fetch the registrar,' said the obstetric house surgeon when he arrived. 'Fetch the senior registrar,' simpered the junior as the procession continued. 'We will have to tell the professor,' said the embryo consultant.

While this trio was glaring at me, the paediatric house physician, an above-average scrum half in his spare time, moved into action. He winkled the baby from the melee, placing it in a small cot on wheels. Running like a man possessed, he headed for the x-ray department.

Meanwhile, the recently delivered Mrs Smythe had abandoned the delights of nitrous oxide and was beginning to surface. The widwife, although still snarling, had recovered sufficient poise to declare that the baby had indeed arrived, but had been taken away for a rest as he had a slight headache!

In those days, delivered mums seemed to have no rights and were usually unable to stand up to people in uniform. The midwife's statement was accepted with a bleary 'What does he weigh?' and 'Will I need stitches?'

Meanwhile, I had been transformed from an apparently normal medical student into a quivering blob of jelly. Beckoned into the corridor by a professoral digit, I almost passed out.

The professor looked stern. 'McGarry, in many years of teaching midwifery, I have never known a medical student to drop a child.' He glanced at the senior registrar. 'I suppose an x-ray will be taken?'

'It has been arranged as a matter of great urgency, sir,' the registrar replied, though he knew full well the idea had never entered his head. In any case, the paediatric department, always an enemy, had snatched the child. It was no longer under obstetric jurisdiction.

The professor decreed that, after the results of the x-ray were known, I was to be the sole bearer of tidings to Mrs Smythe. I was instructed to explain that an accident had happened, that I was entirely to blame, and that I hoped that no subsequent harm was to befall the child.

It was with tears in my eyes that I faced the exhausted mother and did as I had been told. However, on hearing my story, the good lady burst into tears and apologised for being such a burden to me. Astonishingly, she said she hoped I would take up obstetrics permanently. She insisted I was not to blame.

For many years, on each anniversary of this occasion, I received a letter detailing the progress of her son, which has been excellent. Recently, I was told that he had gained a first-class honours degree at one of our better universities, and had been recommended to stay on and do a Ph.D. You know, in a way, I can't help feeling responsible!

REFERENCE
McGarry J 1984 *World Medicine* **19** (October) 39

The Mystery of Byron's Corpse

Byron had, at various times before his death in 1824, expressed wishes to be buried with his dog Bo'sun under the high altar in the ruins of the old priory at Newstead; in his beloved Greece; and, in one of his early poems, among his ancestors.

His friends, particularly John Hobhouse, wanted an Abbey funeral, but this was refused by the Dean and Chapter. The obvious place seemed to be the family vault at the small village, as it then was, of Hucknall Torkard, near Nottingham.

In the little church a final service was held by the parson, the Rev. Charles Nixon, and the vault containing at least 27 members of the Byron family was opened. The remains of the poet were lowered and the vault closed. These remains consisted of the body in a coffin, and an urn containing the heart and brains placed in an oak chest. Thus Byron was brought home to rest with his ancestors. But it was not the end of the story.

Owing to the extravagances of the 6th Lord Byron and his one-man campaigns in Greece, the Byron coffers were sadly depleted. When Captain George Anson Byron succeeded as 7th baron, Newstead had long since been sold and the bulk of what remained of the Byron money had been left to members of the poet's immediate family. Thenceforward no other member of the Byron family was interred in the vault at Hucknall except the poet's daughter, the Countess of Lovelace, whose coffin was deposited there in 1852.

Then, in the 1880s, the little church became inadequate to accommodate the increasing population, so it was almost all taken down and rebuilt. During these alterations the vault was not disturbed structurally but it must have been opened and workmen probably had access to it.

The final chapter in the story of the Byron vault is told by Canon Thomas Gerrard Barber, who was Vicar of Hucknall from 1907 to 1946. The Canon had heard rumours that the body of the poet was not in the family vault at all. So to clear up the point and to determine whether there was, in fact, a crypt under the church (the witnesses to Lady Lovelace's burial said that the vault was arched), he obtained the consent of the Home Office to excavate.

It was on June 15, 1938, that a group of people saw for the first and only time in this century the interior of the Byron vault. It was all done in strict secrecy. Canon Barber rightly guessed that if word got about as to what was afoot, the church would be besieged by what he charitably called 'pilgrims'.

Canon Barber had expected a catacomb with Gothic arches soaring upwards and recesses all around containing the sarcophagi of long-dead Byrons. What he actually saw was a small cramped cell, roughly eight feet high by six feet square with coffins piled untidily one on top of the other, the lower ones having been crushed to dust.

Two of the top coffins, as would be expected, were the last two to be deposited, those of Lord Byron and his daughter, lying almost touching. Either the sightseers at Lady Lovelace's funeral or the workmen who enlarged the church over 30 years later had been busy. Byron's coffin had been opened and the pearls of his coronet resting on it had been stolen. The caps of maintenance inside both Byron's and Lady Lovelace's coronets had gone too, probably also taken as relics.

'Upon closer examination of the coffin' wrote Canon Barber, 'I made the discovery that the lid was loose . . . someone had deliberately opened the coffin.

'A horrible fear came over me that souvenirs might have been taken from within the coffin. The idea was revolting, but I could not dismiss it. Had the body itself been removed? Terrible thought . . .

'Reverently, very reverently, I raised the lid, and before my very eyes lay the embalmed body of Byron in as perfect a condition as when it was placed in the coffin 114 years ago. His features and hair easily recognisable from the portraits with which I was so familiar. The serene, almost happy expression on his face made a profound impression on me . . . I gently lowered the lid of the coffin—and as I did so, breathed a prayer for the peace of his soul.'

Barber's account appeared in 1939. How different from 1824!

Harold Nicholson's book *Byron: The Last Journey* (published to mark the centenary of the poet's death) describes the lying in state at Sir Edward Knatchbull's house in Great George Street, London: 'The room was draped with black and lighted by wax tapers. Mr Hanson [Byron's solicitor] informed Hobhouse that it would be his duty as executor to identify the body.

'Mastering his repulsion, Hobhouse entered the room and gazed upon the coffin. The decaying face that glimmered in the light of the candles was not the face of Byron: Hobhouse was able to identify the body by raising the red velvet pall and glancing at the foot.'

Having read several volumes on the life of Byron during a long convalescence, I went eagerly to Hucknall Torkard for the first time on May 5, 1966. I found a seedy sprawl as unlike the peaceful village of Byron's day as could be imagined. Had the poet returned he would not have recognised any part of it, though he would have viewed with surprise and amusement his statue above the Co-operative store and his name writ large upon the wall of the local cinema.

The church was exciting. Although altered, enlarged and rebuilt almost beyond recognition from its original form, it was dark and mysterious, with a magnificent feeling of space. Victoriana, including some pre-Raphaelite wall mosaics *à la* Burne Jones and fine glass by Kempe, were everywhere.

I learnt from the vicar that there were still one or two people alive who had been present on the day that Canon Barber opened the vault. Among them was Mr James Bettridge, the then caretaker, who lived nearby.

My wife and I eventually met Mr Bettridge, a charming man with great knowledge of the church, and love for it. His description of the vault was more detailed than Canon Barber's. I persuaded him to write it all down, and this is part of his account:

'In early June the Canon informed me that he had received permission from the Home Office to go ahead with the work, and he also invited me to "Come along and lend a hand".

'The date fixed for the opening was June 15, 1938. All were bound to secrecy, to forestall undesirable sightseers. Accordingly, on that lovely summer's afternoon, Mr J. C. Woodsend, a mason from Nottingham, and three of his workmen, arrived at the rear of the church with a lorry containing picks, shovels, planks etc. and work began.

'Old prints show that the entrance to the vault was covered by two large flagstones into which four iron rings were fastened. One of these stones is visible, the second one is now covered by the chancel steps. The masons—directed by Mr Woodsend—soon got to work with hammers and chisels, breaking the tiles around the stone, then the

216

lower chancel step was removed and both stones were lifted. We could then see the interior of the vault.

'To everyone's disappointment the vault was found to measure a mere seven-and-a-half feet by six feet. The coffins were piled one on top of each other, in three stacks; on the left the Lords, in the centre the Ladies and on the right a few children.

'After Mr Lane [the diocesan surveyor] had made measurements of the vault and staircase, closer examination of the coffins began.

'The uppermost coffins of the first and second stacks were of striking appearance, being of oak. That on the left bore a coronet from which the cap of maintenance and pearls were missing, as also were the name-plates and some of the coffin handles. The coffin below this was in rather poor condition, the wood having decayed, leaving part of the leaden coffin exposed. The third one was entirely lead and had already lost its shape, having been crushed by those above. Lower still all the coffins were flattened.

'The floor of the vault was covered to a depth of eight or nine inches in debris, consisting of dust, decayed wood, pieces of lead and numerous bones. All this debris must have been the remains of the early burials.

'Later, Canon Barber decided to make a closer examination of what we were pretty certain was the poet's coffin. The oak lid was found to be loose, and raising it we could see the lead shell which had been cut open. Inside this leaden case was a wooden coffin, the lid of which had never been fastened.

'After some deliberation, Canon Barber very reverently raised the lid, and suddenly I gazed upon the face of Lord Byron . . . The features, with the slightly protruding lower lip and the mass of curly hair, were easily recognisable from the many pictures we had seen. The body had been covered but the funerary clothing had decayed.

'The head was slightly raised as though it had rested on a pillow; parts of which could still be seen in the corners of the coffin. The colour of the body was dark stone. Both feet seemed to be normal. The right foot, however, had been severed just above the ankle, and lay in the corner of the coffin. I heard afterwards that in the doctor's opinion this was a skilful amputation made after death; and the cause of the poet's lameness was a deformed Achilles tendon. Neither foot was clubbed. The vault was finally sealed on the following day.'

There is a question to be answered as a result of all this. Why could Byron's closest friend apparently not recognise him soon after his death and yet 114 years later a number of rational and intelligent people gave evidence of recognising a face already familiar to them through portraits?

Was it a question of auto-suggestion? Did they recognise Byron

217

because they *wanted* to recognise him? The real test would have been to confront a third person with the visage—someone who had not the faintest idea beforehand. We shall never know now.

Lord Byron. (Courtesy Mansell Collection.)

Canon Barber seemed sure and the late Mr Bettridge was in no doubt whatever. What a pity that Mr Bullock, the photographer, did not take a photograph of Byron. It would have been easy, but Canon Barber thought it a very irreverent thing to do, so photographs were confined to coffins and coffin plates. Mr Bettridge's family had lived in Hucknall since the time of Lord Byron, and he remembered his grand-mother telling him how she had seen the funeral of Byron's daughter Lady Lovelace in 1852, and his great grandmother had seen the cortège of Byron himself.

To have gazed upon the face of Lord Byron must have been an uncanny but highly privileged occasion. Apart from an admittedly morbid appeal, such experiences bridge time effortlessly and bring us nearer to our forebears. The past suddenly becomes the present as the fog of history rises for a moment and we are dazzled by the light.

218

REFERENCE
Innes-Smith R *Sunday Telegraph* 7 February 1988

Bathtub Elixir puts Estonian behind Bars

You can't be a profit-maker in your own official basement—that was the lesson learned by an Estonian biochemist when he concocted a cure-all 'health elixir'. The biochemist was arrested last December, but details of his bizarre case have only just been made public—and investigations are still continuing.

I Khint, a citizen of Tallin, capital of the Soviet republic, installed several large bathtubs in the depths of the Special Design and Technological Bureau, of which he was director, and brewed and sold large quantities of his quack drink, making a handsome profit—before he was arrested.

The ingredients of the concoction were rather likes those of Macbeth's witches' cauldron: pigs' feet, blood and entrails, mushrooms, beets, cabbage, dandelion, carrots, nettles, sugar and a 'secret fermentation' formula. After being strained, the liquid was bottled for sale to eager consumers.

Though the contents were neither analysed nor officially approved, Khint managed to talk the Soviet Ministry of Health into giving him a permit to sell his 'Health Elixir' at a 'middle ceiling price'. The elixir was widely recommended as a panacea for every malady—including cancer.

The enterprising Khint organised seminars, conferences, and lectures to promote his elixir. He even managed to attract the interest of the Soviet State Planning Commission by claiming that when the elixir was diluted in the drinking water of livestock, productivity increased from 20–40 per cent.

Khint's come-uppance came when the medical authorities finally checked his concoction and determined that it was toxic, addictive and devoid of medical value. He and his numerous accomplices were tried and convicted on a string of charges. Khint got a maximum 15-year sentence.

REFERENCE
The Sunday Times May 13 1984

Capgras Syndrome

People who believe that a relative or close friend has been replaced by their double are said to suffer from Capgras Syndrome. While these delusions can be devastating and emotionally hurtful for the relative, they are not usually in any danger.

However, a report in the *British Journal of Psychiatry* contains a chilling account from a secure psychiatric unit in Missouri. A man there accused his step-father of being a robot and subsequently decapitated him to look for batteries and microfilm inside his head.

REFERENCE
The *Independent* 23 February 1988

French X-Ray Finds a Screw Loose

It was reported from Cannes that doctors could scarcely believe their eyes when a routine x-ray of a man complaining of headaches showed a seven inch screwdriver embedded in his skull.

On further investigation they found the tool was not in the man's head—but in the x-ray machine where it had been left by a careless technician.

REFERENCE
London Evening Standard 22 February 1985

Self-Inflicted Frontal Lobotomy

Brain surgery which can change people's personalities or behaviour has had a controversial history. Until high-powered scanners made it easier to make tiny and accurate incisions in the tissue, the success of operations was hit and miss.

A bizarre tale in the *British Journal of Psychiatry* describes a 19-year-old man who had suffered for years from severe compulsive and obsessive behaviour. He became increasingly depressed and attempted to commit suicide by shooting himself in the mouth. He survived the injuries but coincidentally performed a precise operation on the frontal lobes of his brain: when he eventually recovered from his ordeal his ritualistic behaviour was much less pronounced.

REFERENCE

The *Independent* 20 January 1988

Almost-failed EEC Contraception

(Contributed by Mr J M McGarry, FRCOG, Barnstaple.)

Prior to their marriage contraception had been by the sheath (now more contemporaneously called the condom). Although their premarital sexual activity had been reasonably satisfying to both partners, a decision was taken during the pre-nuptual preparation that she would better be fitted with a diaphragm. It being 1961, when the Pill had only just come on to the market, the choice of oral contraception was not made because in that immediate post-thalidomide era this young couple wanted to wait until the new 'pill' had been tested by time. In any case the low risk of pregnancy when using the cap and spermicides was one that the espoused were prepared to take.

After the wedding breakfast they hurriedly left for a honeymoon that was to be taken exploring the Mosel valley in Germany as they both had oenophilic interests and this seemed to be a good opportunity to combine several pleasures at the same time. The Weymouth–Cherbourg ferry crossing was rough so the first night in France did not involve any love-making. The next day's drive across France to the Luxembourg border was similarly exhausting: so marital bliss was again postponed. In a cafe in Longwy in eastern France a late coffee was followed by a trip to the Ladies room. Here she truly 'powdered her nose', her powder compact being similar to the plastic case containing the contraceptive cap. Owing to tiredness and hurry something was left in front of the mirror in the 'Ladies'.

Their open-topped Morris soon crossed into Luxembourg. Passports were duly stamped with Gallic indifference by both sets of Customs and in that late evening one of the smallest countries of the world was quickly traversed, a distance of 45 km. The Luxembourg/German border was crossed with Prussian efficiency and they were soon ensconced in a Mosel valley hotel inside Germany. A suitable honeymoon repast was washed down with Bernkastel and they retired early to bed.

Just as his undressed unrequited loins were beginning to tingle she gasped that she had lost her cap. Memories of the shelf in front of the mirror in the Ladies in the cafe in Longwy quickly dawned and with a sigh he set out to traverse Luxembourg for the second time that evening. Each set of Customs examined his passport with greater diligence this time but he was eventually let through.

On arrival at the French cafe it was of course shut. An irate Patron was roused from his slumbers, and a request to go into the ladies 'loo' was reluctantly acceded to. Fortunately there was the plastic case and its contents intact and undamaged. It was hastily pocketed and with profuse apologies to the cafe owner the luckless groom prepared to cross Luxembourg for the third time in one day.

The Customs officers by now had become increasingly suspicious and during the next four hours his person and car were rigorously searched by four different sets of Customs officers. All they found was his passport and a Dutch Cap. Each time the cap was discovered he tried to explain in halting schoolboy French and German the reason for it being on his person.

The Mosel valley hotel was eventually reached at 4 am. Our frustrated suitor had to wake up the owner of the small hostelry who was not amused; this time with German bad grace instead of French.

He crawled into bed clutching the cased cap. Unfortunately the lady's unfamiliar sampling of the Bernkastel had induced a deep soporiferous state. Also his phenomenal achievement of becoming the first person to completely cross the same country three times in one day (albeit a small country) had so exhausted him that amorous cavorting did not seem to be worth the effort.

The marriage was consummated on the fourth day and both considered it was worth waiting for. At conventions of French, German and Luxembourg Customs officers, the antics of this strange English doctor in the open car are still talked about with unbelieving awe. No wonder it took us so long to get into the EEC.

Premature Burial

In some instances simulation of death has been so exact that it has led to premature internment. There are many such cases on record[1] and it is a popular superstition that all the gruesome tales of persons buried alive and returning to life, only to find themselves hopelessly lost in a narrow coffin many feet below the surface of the earth, are true.

222

Indeed, because of this dread by members of the public, doctors for generations have been denounced for their inability to discover an infallible sign of death. There was even a suggestion in the *Scientific American* of 1896[3] that x-rays could be used for this purpose:

Dead flesh offers more resistance to the penetration of the rays than living, and a glance at the radiograph of the person would determine whether it was that of a corpse or not.

Most of the instances of premature burial on record, and particularly those from lay journals, are vivid exaggerations, drawn possibly from such trivial signs as a corpse found with a fist tightly clenched or a face distorted—which are the inspiration of the horrible details of the dying struggles of the person in the coffin. However, in all modern methods of burial, even if life were not extinct, there could be no possibility of consciousness or of struggling. Absolute asphyxiation would soon follow the closing of the coffin lid. Nevertheless, mistakes have been made, particularly in the instances of catalepsy or trance, and during epidemics of fevers and plagues, in which there was an absolute necessity of hasty burial for the prevention of contagion. It is also said that Vesalius, sometimes called the Father of Anatomy, having been sent for to perform an autopsy on a woman subject to hysterical convulsions, and who was supposed to be dead, on making the first incision perceived by her movements and cries that she was still alive. This circumstance becoming known, it rendered him so odious that he had to leave the community in which he practiced, and it is believed that he never entirely recovered from the shock it gave him.

It is probably far more likely that any stories of a return to life which are true, are those when the event occurred after certification of death but before burial. One such event[2] has been related to me by an impeccable source, a health services correspondent of a well known paper who was the daughter of the Irish GP who was an eyewitness:

The GP had pronounced one of his patients dead and the usual arrangements were made for the wake. The GP was invited and, there they all were—the family of the dead man, the priest, the district nurse, *et al*, all taking their place around the scrubbed clean kitchen table on which Patrick lay in his open coffin. The whisky and the porter flowed freely: the mood grew merrier and merrier as they celebrated the arrival of the dear departed soul at the pearly gates. Then suddenly, the 'corpse' sat up, assessed the situation and asked 'Is this a private party, or can anyone join in?'. On being given the facts, the poor man had a coronary and dropped dead. The wake continued from where it had briefly left off and in due course Patrick was buried and sent on his heavenly way.

REFERENCES
[1] Gould G M and Pyle W L 1900 *Anomalies and Curiosities of Medicine* (Philadelphia: Saunders)
[2] Harding M 1984 Personal communication
[3] Mould R F 1980 'X-ray mystery' *BIR Bulletin* **6** No 4

Yellow Fever Experiment in Cuba

In 1900 there was an epidemic of yellow fever among the US troops stationed in Havana after the Spanish–American war. Fifteen years earlier it had been suggested by Charles Finlay[1] that mosquitoes carried the disease from man to man, but this had been largely ignored and the US Secretary of War appointed a four-man medical board of Walter Reed and three assistants, Carroll, Agramonte and Lazear, 'to pursue scientific investigations with reference to the infectious disease prevalent on the island of Cuba.[2] Following the theory of Finlay, they hatched mosquitoes from eggs, induced the insects to bite patients with known yellow fever and then maintained colonies of presumably infected mosquitoes for experiments. Some of these bit Carroll, Lazear and a volunteer from the US Army, Private Dean, and all contracted yellow fever. Carroll and Dean recovered but unfortunately Lazear died. However, it had been shown that mosquitoes carried the disease from man to man.

Final proof that yellow fever was transmitted only by mosquito bite came when three other volunteers never exposed to Cuban mosquitoes slept for 20 nights in a room free of mosquitoes, but full of mattresses, pillows, towels, sheets, underwear, pyjamas and blankets soiled with blood and a variety of discharges from known yellow fever patients. None of the volunteers became sick.

REFERENCES
[1] Finlay C 1886 'Yellow fever: its transmission by means of the culex mosquito' *Am. J. Med. Sci.* **92** 395–409
[2] Comroe J H 1977 *Retrospectroscope* (Von Gehr Press: Menlo Park, CA)

Vaccination

Dr Edward Jenner's 1796 discovery of vaccination, the immunisation for smallpox, is well known. What is not so well known are the following anecdotes:

The first child to be vaccinated in Russia was named Vaccinov and educated at the expense of the nation as a tribute to the discovery.

During the 1870–1 Franco-Prussian War, vaccination was compulsory in the Prussian army where only 297 died of smallpox. It was not compulsory in the French army and 23 400 died from smallpox. The French also lost the war!

The first vaccination. Edward Jenner inoculating an eight-year-old boy, James Phipps, with cow pox matter on 14 May 1796. (Courtesy Mansell Collection.)

A Deaf Australian Magistrate

A slightly deaf Magistrate had just heard a case of larceny, to which the defendant had pleaded guilty. The Prosecutor had read out a long list of prior convictions for dishonesty, assaults and resisting arrests. The Magistrate then asked the defendant, who was unrepresented by Counsel, if he had anything to say in extenuation. The defendant said, 'Bugger all'.

The Magistrate did not hear what the defendant said and he leaned over the Bench and whispered to the Clerk of Sessions, sitting immediately below and in front of him and said, 'What did he say?'

The Clerk said, 'Bugger all'.

The Magistrate said, 'That's funny, I could have sworn I saw his lips move'.

REFERENCE
Gillespie-Jones A S 1978 *The Lawyer Who Laughed* (Hutchinson of Australia: Richmond, Australia) p. 141

Sir Anthony Oyster

In the late 1830s *The Lancet* was looking for any evidence of abuse of power or inefficiency in the hospitals of the day. The blow fell on the Westminster Hospital surgeon Sir Anthony Carlisle, President of the Royal College of Surgeons in 1828 and 1837, and a pupil of John Hunter. He had delivered the 1820 Hunter Oration at the Royal College, taking as his title *The Anatomy of the Oyster*.

Sir Anthony Carlisle FRS, Surgeon to Westminster Hospital, 1793–1840.

226

Thomas Walkley, the editor of *The Lancet* attacked Carlisle, calling him Sir Anthony Oyster, on the subject of a man called Thomas Holmes, admitted to Westminster Hospital with an injured arm, and who subsequently developed delirium tremens. Sir Anthony had not seen him on admission to hospital, but passing through the wards some days later he noticed that Holmes was in delirium and was causing discomfort to the other patients. Thereupon he signed a certificate of insanity which he left with the House Surgeon so that if necessary, and if the patient needed it, the certificate could be signed by a second medical man and the patient could then be removed as insane.

A subsequent enquiry by the Board of Governors established that the patient was a heavy drinker, had had previous attacks and that the certificate was supplied by Sir Anthony at the request of the Chairman of the Board's investigating committee, who had previously ordered Holmes to be put in a straitjacket.

Further evidence showed where *The Lancet* had got its story: from the hospital Apothecary and the House Surgeon. The former rather ingenuously said 'Our only object in publishing was to preserve an instance of the efficiency of large doses of opium in the treatment of delirium tremens' but also added that the Board must now consider Carlisle's fitness for hospital duties.

Sir Anthony was exonerated, but one year later *The Lancet* published an account of a surgical round by Carlisle which rather ridiculed the old gentleman, written by one Clarke. Carlisle was annoyed by this since he had not realised that Clarke had attended the round for such journalistic purposes and told his medical students that if they ever saw Clarke in the hospital again he would be obliged if they would 'rough handle him a little'. When Clarke was told of this, he paid a fee and became a Governor of Westminster Hospital.

However, at his first Board meeting he was recognised and had to jab the point of his umbrella into the eye of one student in order to escape to the Board Room. Then, after the meeting the students pursued Clarke with so much fury that he was forced to take refuge in a local public house.

Sir Anthony Carlisle died in 1840 but Clarke remained a member of the Board of Governors at least until 1845 with Board meetings continuing to be stormy and Clarke (by then an Assistant Editor of *The Lancet*) suggesting that the hospital must have been built over the old Westminster Cockpit!

REFERENCE
Humble J G and Hansell P 1974 *Westminster Hospital, 1716–1974* 2nd edn (London: Pitman Medical)

The Birth of Anaesthesia

(By permission of Professor Harold Ellis.)

If I were asked to name the most dramatic moment in surgery, it would not be when the clamps were taken off the first heart transplant, nor the first esophagectomy, or the ablation of any other major organ but a very simple, almost trivial affair—the removal of a benign tumour of the neck. The date was October 16, 1846, the place was Massachusetts General Hospital in Boston, and the event was the watershed between the past agonies of surgery and the modern era, now only a little over a century old, when patients enjoy the blissful oblivion of anesthesia.

William Morton, the dentist who was to become the father of modern anesthesia, was twenty-seven years of age. He had been experimenting with ether for dental extractions, and his first patient, Eben Frost, had a tooth pulled out under the influence of ether saturated into a handkerchief on September 30, 1846. The patient testifies as follows:

> This is to certify that I applied to Dr Morton at 9 o'clock this evening suffering under the most violent toothache; that Dr Morton took out his pocket handkerchief, saturated with a preparation of his, from which I breathed for about half a minute, and then was lost in sleep. In an instant more I awoke and saw my tooth lying upon the floor. I did not experience the slightest pain whatever. I remained 20 minutes in his office afterward, and felt no unpleasant effects from the operation.

Dr H J Bigelow, son of the great Jacob Bigelow, was attracted by the newspaper reports of Morton's work and went to see him. Impressed by what he saw, he introduced Morton to Professor John Collins Warren, then sixty-eight years of age and one of the country's leading surgeons. A few days later Morton received the following letter:

> I write at the request of Dr John Collins Warren to invite you to be present Friday morning, October 16, at 10 o'clock at the hospital to administer to a patient who is then to be operated upon, the preparation you have invented to diminish the sensibility to pain.

The letter was signed by Dr C F Heywood, House Surgeon.

It was now only two weeks since ether had been administered to Frost, but already Morton had progressed from a soaked handkerchief to a simple anesthetic machine. This consisted of a two-necked glass globe, one neck allowing the inflow of air, the other fitted with a wooden mouthpiece through which the patient inhaled air across the

228

surface of the ether in the bottom of the jar.

All the anxieties of a great clinical trial are summed up by Morton's young wife, who wrote:

> The night before the operation my husband worked until 1 or 2 o'clock in the morning upon his inhaler. I assisted him, nearly beside myself with anxiety, for the strongest influences had been brought to bear upon me to dissuade him from making this attempt. I had been told that one of two things was sure to happen; either the test would fail and my husband would be ruined by the world's ridicule, or he would kill the patient and be tried for manslaughter. Thus I was drawn in two ways; for while I had bounded confidence in my husband, it did not seem possible that so young a man could be wiser than the learned and scientific men before whom he proposed to make his demonstration.

The operating theatre at the Massachusetts General Hospital was situated just below the central dome of the old building. It is preserved to this day. On the morning of October 16, it was crowded with surgeons and medical students. The audience included both Jacob Bigelow and his son, Henry. The patient was Gilbert Abbott, twenty years of age, who had a benign vascular tumor of the neck. Petrified at the thought of the pain of his operation, he had readily agreed to the experiment. Professor Warren explained to the audience how much he had always wished to free his patients from the pain of operation and for that reason had agreed to the experiment. The time of the operation arrived and passed. By ten minutes past ten Professor Warren picked up his knife and said 'As Dr Morton has not arrived, I presume he is otherwise engaged.' (I personally believe that this was simply Morton creating a tradition, which has been handed down from one generation of anesthetists to another, of keeping the surgeon waiting.)

Just as Abbott was being strapped down on the operating chair, a breathless and flustered Morton arrived; he had been modifying his apparatus up to the very last moment. Warren said, 'Well, sir, your patient is ready.'

'Are you afraid?' Morton asked the patient. 'No, I feel confident that I will do precisely what you tell me.' Morton applied his ether, the smell heavily disguised with some aromatic agent to prevent people from recognizing it and discovering its secret. Turning to Warren, Morton was now able to say, '*Your* patient is ready, doctor.' Many years later Mrs Morton described the scene:

> Then in all parts of the ampitheatre there came a quick catching of breath, followed by silence almost deathlike, as Dr Warren stepped forward and prepared to operate. . . . The patient lay silent, with eyes closed as if in sleep; but everyone present fully expected to hear a shriek of agony ring out as the knife struck down into the sensitive nerves,

but the stroke came with no accompanying cry. Then another and another, and still the patient lay silent, sleeping while the blood from the severed artery spurted forth. The surgeon was doing his work, and the patient was free from pain.

The operation took thirty minutes, and at the end Abbott agreed that the whole affair had been free from pain. Warren turned to the audience and said, 'Gentlemen, this is no humbug.' It took a few moments before the sensational importance of what they had seen struck the audience, who then rushed forward to congratulate Morton, to examine the patient, and to ask him over and over again if the operation really had been painless. Everyone in that room must have realized that they had witnessed an historic occasion.

William Morton making the first demonstration of etherisation at the Massachusetts General Hospital, surrounded by the medical staff of that institution 16 October 1846 (Courtesy Mansell Collection.)

It was now necessary to proceed to the crucial experiment. The new agent might be effective in the removal of a subcutaneous lump from the neck, but would it work in a capital operation, an amputation? A case was duly scheduled, therefore, for November 7. Before this could be put to the test, a burning ethical issue arose. Should Morton be allowed to administer a secret agent, beneficial though it might be, or should its use be prohibited until its nature was revealed to the medical profession? Warren was prepared to go ahead, his only concern being relief of pain, but the Massachusetts Medical Society

230

resolved unanimously—no formula, no patients. Even though Morton offered to supply the preparation free for use in the Boston hospitals, the doctors remained adamant.

On the very day of the operation the argument continued, with the patient waiting in the anteroom and the theatre packed to the ceiling with expectant doctors and students. Unable to bear the thought of the patient's suffering, Morton quietly announced that his liquid was indeed sulfuric ether.

The patient was a twenty-one-year-old servant girl, Alice Mohan, who had been in the hospital since the previous March with tuberculosis of the knee joint. Dr George Hayward was to perform the amputation, with Warren and Bigelow in attendance. Morton administered the ether, and after some coughing, the patient fell into a deep sleep. Hayward stuck a pin into her arm and, when there was no reaction, rapidly amputated her leg. As he finished, Alice began to groan and move. Hayward bent over her and said, 'I guess you've been asleep, Alice.' 'I think I have, sir,' she replied. 'Well, you know why we brought you here; are you ready?' 'Yes sir, I am ready.' Hayward then reached down, picked up the amputated limb from the sawdust, showed it to her and said, 'It's all done, Alice.' (What Alice said when she saw her leg has not been recorded.)

Scenes of intense excitement were then seen, with the medical audience clapping and shouting with amazement. Morton described the affair modestly: 'I administered the ether with perfect success. This was the first case of amputation.' The patient did well and was discharged from the hospital in time for Christmas.

News of 'the most glorious, nay, the most god-like discovery of this or any other age' spread with amazing speed. Bigelow wrote a letter on November 28 to Dr Francis Boott, an American friend living in Gower Street, London, near the University College Hospital. He enclosed a copy of his son's account of the details of the operations and Morton's apparatus. Boott in turn conveyed the news to Robert Liston, Professor of Surgery at University College Hospital, London, and Liston got his colleague, Dr William Squire, to obtain ether from an uncle of his, who had a chemist's shop on Oxford Street. The apparatus was assembled, and on December 19, Squire anesthetized Boott's niece for a dental extraction carried out by James Robinson. The operation was uneventful, and plans were made for major surgery two days later.

The patient was Frederick Churchill, a butler who had been admitted a month previously with chronic osteomyelitis of the tibia. At two o'clock the operating theatre at the Univeristy College Hospital was packed to capacity. Squire called for a volunteer among the doctors and medical students present, saying that he had only tried the apparatus once before and would like one more rehearsal before submitting a patient to its influence for a capital operation. No one moved. The theatre porter, Shelldrake, was therefore asked to submit to the test. He was not a good choice to try out an anesthetic as he was fat, plethoric, and with a liver no doubt very used to strong liquor. After a few deep breaths of ether, Shelldrake leaped off the table and ran out of the room, cursing Squire and everybody else at the top of his voice.

Fifteen minutes later, Liston arrived, and Churchill was brought into the theatre by the now sober and recovered Shelldrake. Squire now took the precaution of choosing two hefty students to stand by in case the patient repeated the porter's performance. What happened next has been brilliantly described by Dr F W Cock:

A firm step is heard, and Robert Liston enters—that magnificent figure of a man, six foot two inches in height, with a most commanding expression of countenance. He nods quietly to Squire and, turning round to the packed crowd of onlookers, students, colleagues, old students and many of the neighbouring practitioners, says somewhat dryly, 'We are going to try a Yankee dodge to-day, gentlemen, for making men insensible.' He then takes from a long narrow case one of the straight amputating knives of his own invention. It is evidently a favourite instrument, for on the handle are little notches showing the number of times he had used it before. . . . The patient is carried in on the stretcher and laid on the table. The tube is put into his mouth, William Squire holds it at the patient's nostrils. A couple of dressers stand by, to hold the patient if necessary, but he never moves and blows and gurgles away quite quietly. William Squire looks at Liston and says, 'I think he will do, sir.' 'Take the artery, Mr Cadge,' cries Liston. Ransome, the House Surgeon, holds the limb. 'Now gentle-men, time me,' he says to the students. A score of watches are pulled out in reply. A huge left hand grasps the thigh, a thrust of the long, straight knife, two or three rapid sawing movements, and the upper flap is made; under go his fingers, and the flap is held back; another thrust, and the point of the knife comes out in the angle of the upper flap; two or three more lightning-like movements and the lower flap is cut, under goes the great thumb and holds it back also; the dresser, holding the saw by its end, yields it to the surgeon and takes the knife in return—half a dozen strokes, and Ransome places the limb in the sawdust, 'Twenty-eight seconds,' says William Squire. The femoral artery is taken upon a tenaculum and tied with two stout ligatures, and five or six more vessels with the bow forceps and single thread, a strip of wet lint put between the flaps, and the stump dressed. The patient, trying to raise himself, says, 'When are you going to begin? Take me back, I can't have it done.' He is shown the elevated stump, drops back and weeps a little; then the porters come in and he is taken back to bed. Five minutes have elapsed since he left it. As he goes out, Liston turns again to his audience, so excited that he almost stammers and hesitates, and exclaims, 'This Yankee dodge, gentlemen, beats mesmerism hollow.'

Liston could hardly have realized at that moment that the need for rapid surgery, which his skill had brought to such a pitch of perfection, was now to be replaced by the new era, when anesthesia would allow calm and unhurried operations.

Immediately after Christmas, ether anaesthesia reached Westminster Hospital, two or three miles down the road. The operation, however, was far less grand—the scraping off of some venereal warts from a lady of doubtful reputation.

As for Morton, the rest of his short life was not a happy one, although he had the compensation of using ether with great success during the American Civil War. He died in 1868 at only forty-eight years of age. The citizens of Boston erected a monument over his grave, the inscription on which was composed by Dr Jacob Bigelow:

Inventor and revealer of anaesthetic inhalation
By whom pain in surgery was averted and annulled
Before whom in all time surgery was agony
Since whom science has controlled the pain.

REFERENCES
Ellis H 1984 *Famous Operations* (Harwal Publishing Co.: Media, PA) pp 51–61
Cock F W 1915 'The first major operation under ether in England' *Am. J. Surg.* **29** (Suppl) 98
Coltart D J 1972 'Surgery between Hunter and Lister as exemplified by the life and works of Robert Liston (1794–1847)' *Proc. R. Soc. Med.* **65** 556
MacQuitty B 1969 *The Battle for Oblivion. Discovery of Anaesthesia* (Harrap: London)
Warren J C 1897 'The influence of anaesthesia on the surgery of the nineteenth century' *Trans. Am. Surg. Assoc.* **15** 1

Florence Nightingale as Medical Statistician, 1859–61

Few books made a greater impression on Miss Nightingale than those of Adolphe Quetelet, the Belgian astronomer, meteorologist, and statistician; and she had few friends whom she valued more highly than Dr William Farr, the leading statistician of her day in this country. From his meteorological studies, Quetelet deduced a law of the flowering of plants. One of his cases was the lilac. The common lilac flowers, according to Quetelet's law, when the sum of the squares of the mean daily temperatures, counted from the end of the frosts, equals 4264° centigrade. Miss Nightingale was greatly interested in such calculations, and the lilac had a special place in her year. Lady Verney's birthday was April 19, and a branch of flowering lilac was Florence's regular birthday present to her sister. Miss Nightingale used to talk of Quetelet's law with great delight, and commended it to gardening friends for verification in their Naturalist's Diaries. But this is a lighter example of Quetelet's researches. What fascinated Miss Nightingale most was his *Essai de physique sociale*, in which he showed the possibility of applying the statistical method to social dynamics, and deduced from such method various conclusions with regard to the physical and intellectual qualities of man. In regard to sanitation, we have heard already of the reforms which Miss Nightingale was instrumental in carrying out in Army Medical Statistics. She turned next to the question of Hospital Statistics, where improvement seemed desirable both for the surer advance of medical knowledge and in the interests of good administration.

THE CRIMEAN WAR

Miss Nightingale had been painfully impressed during the Crimean War with the statistical carelessness which prevailed in the military hospitals. Even the number of deaths was not accurately recorded. 'At Scutari,' she said, 'three separate registers were kept. First, the Adjutant's daily Head-roll of soldiers' burials, on which it may be presumed no one was entered who was not buried, although it is possible that some may have been buried who were not entered. Second, the Medical Officers' Return, in regard to which it is quite certain that hundreds of men were buried who never appeared upon it. Third, the return made in the Orderly Room, which is only remarkable as giving a totally different account of the deaths from either of the others.' When Miss Nightingale came home, and began examining Hospital Statistics in London, she found, not indeed such glaring carelessness as this, but a complete lack of scientific co-ordination. The statistics of hospitals were kept on no uniform plan. Each hospital followed its own nomenclature and classification of diseases. There had been no reduction on any uniform model of the vast amount of observations which had been made. 'So far as relates,' she said, 'either to medical or to sanitary science, these observations in their present state bear exactly the same relation as an indefinite number of astronomical observations made without concert, and reduced to no common standard, would bear to the progress of astronomy.'

234

MODEL FORMS

Miss Nightingale set herself to remedy this defect. With assistance from friendly doctors on the medical side, and of Dr Farr, of the Registrar-General's Office, on the statistical, she prepared (1) a standard list, under various Classes and Orders, of diseases, and (2) model Hospital Statistical Forms. The general adoption of her Forms would, as she wrote, 'enable us to ascertain the relative mortality in different hospitals, as well as of different diseases and injuries at the same and at different ages, the relative frequency of different diseases and injuries among the classes which enter hospitals in different countries, and in different districts of the same countries.' Then, again, the relation of the duration of cases to the general utility of a hospital had never been shown. Miss Nightingale's proposed forms 'would enable the mortality in hospitals, and also the mortality from particular diseases, injuries, and operations, to be ascertained with accuracy; and these facts, together with the duration of cases, would enable the value of particular methods of treatment and of special operations to be brought to statistical proof. The sanitary state of the hospital itself could likewise be ascertained.' Having formed her plan, Miss Nightingale proceeded with her usual resourcefulness to action. She had her Model Forms printed (1859), and she persuaded some of the London hospitals to adopt them experimentally. Sir James Paget at St Bartholomew's was particularly helpful; St Mary's, St Thomas's, and University College also agreed to use the Forms. She and Dr Farr studied the results, which were sufficient to show how large a field for statistical analysis and inquiry would be opened by the general adoption of her Forms.

The case was now ready for a further move. Dr Farr was one of the General Secretaries of the International Statistical Congress which was to meet in London in the summer of 1860. He and Miss Nightingale drew up the programme for the Second Section of the Congress (Sanitary Statistics), and her scheme for Uniform Hospital Statistics was the principal subject of discussion. Her Model Forms were printed, with an explanatory memorandum; the Section discussed and approved them, and a resolution was passed that her proposals should be communicated to all the Governments represented at the Congress. She took a keen interest in all the proceedings, and gave a series of breakfast-parties, presided over by her cousin Hilary, to the delegates, some of whom were afterwards admitted to the presence of their hostess upstairs. The foreign delegates much appreciated this courtesy, as their spokesman said at the closing meeting of the Congress; 'all the world knows the name of Miss Nightingale,' and it was an honour to be received by 'the illustrious invalid, the

Providence of the English Army.' The written instructions sent by 'the Providence' to her cousin for the entertainment of the guests show her care for little things and her knowledge of the weaknesses of great men: 'Take care that the cream for breakfast is not turned.' 'Put back Dr. X's big book where he can see it when drinking his tea.' Miss Nightingale also induced her friend Mrs. Herbert to invite the statisticians to an evening party. The feast of statistics acted upon her as a tonic. 'She has been more than usually ill for the last four or five weeks,' wrote her cousin Hilary; 'now I cannot help thinking that her strength is rallying a little; she is much interested in the Statistical Congress.' Congresses, like wars, are sometimes 'muddled through' by our country, and Miss Nightingale was able here and there to smooth ruffled plumes. A distinguished friend of hers, though his name had been printed as one of the secretaries of a Section, had not received so much as an intimation of the place of meeting; he was disgusted at so unbusiness-like an omission, and was half inclined to sulk in his tents. Miss Nightingale's letter on the subject is characteristic:—

(*Miss Nightingale to Dr T Graham Balfour*) 30 OLD BURLINGTON ST., *July* 12 [1860]. You are quite right in what you say. We are all of us in the same boat. And, if it were not that England *would not be* the mercantile nation she *is*, if she had not business habits somewhere, I should wonder from my experience where they are. Certain of us, who were asked to do business for the Statistical Congress, had it all ready since December last—and were not able to get it out of the Registrar-General's Office till this week. Certain of us were asked to do business this morning, and to have it ready by to-night, which if *not* done, would arrest the proceedings of the Congress, and *if* done, must be the fruit of only five hours' consideration, when five months might just as well have been granted for it. I don't say this is so bad as the treatment of you who are Secretary. But still it is provoking to see a great International business worked in this way.

What I want now is to put a good face upon it before the foreigners. Let *them* not see our short-comings and disunions. Many countries, far behind us in political business, are far before us in organization-power. If any one has ever been behind the scenes, living in the interior, of the Maison Mère of the 'Sisters of Charity' at Paris, as I have—and seen their Counting House and Office, all worked by women—an Office which has twelve thousand Officials (all women) scattered all over the known world—an office to compare with which, in business habits, I have never seen any, either Government or private, in England—they will think, like me, that it is this mere business-power which keeps these enormous religious 'orders' going.

I hope that you will try to impress these foreign Delegates, then, with a sense of *our* 'enormous business-power' (in which I don't believe one bit), and to keep the Congress going. Many thanks for all your papers. I trust you will settle some sectional business with the Delegates here to-morrow morning. And I trust I shall be able to see you, if not to-morrow morning, soon.

Mind, I don't mean anything against *your* Office by this tirade. On the contrary, I believe it is one of the few efficient ones now in existence.

Florence Nightingale, 1858.

Having received the *imprimatur* of an International Congress, Miss Nightingale circulated her paper on Hospital Statistics widely among medical men and hospital officials. Thereby she produced immediate effect. She printed large quantities of her Model Forms, and supplied them, on request, to hospitals in various parts of the country. Through the good offices of M. Mohl, she also worked upon public opinion in France. 'Some months ago,' she wrote to Dr Farr (Oct. 20, 1860), 'I got inserted into the leading medical journals of Paris an article on the proposed Hospital Registers; and you see they are at work.' the London hospitals took the matter up. Guy's printed a statistical analysis of its cases from 1854 to 1861; St Thomas's, of its from 1857 to 1860; St Bartholomews, a table of its cases for 1860. With regard to the future, a meeting was held at Guy's Hospital on June 21, 1861, and it was unanimously agreed—by delegates from Guy's, St Bartholomew's, St Thomas's, the London, St George's, King's College, the Middlesex, and St Mary's—that the Metropolitan Hospitals should adopt one uniform system of Registration of Patients; that each hospital should publish its statistics annually, and that Miss Nightingale's Model Forms should as far as possible be adopted. She called further attention to her scheme in a paper sent to the Social Science Congress at Dublin in August 1861, and incorporated it in a later edition of her *Notes on Hospitals*. The statistics of the various hospitals which had accepted her Forms were published in the *Journal of the Statistical Society* for September 1862, but I do not find that the experiment has been continued. So far from there being any uniform hospital statistics, of the kind contemplated by Miss Nightingale, even in London some of the hospitals do not keep, or at any rate do not publish, any at all. The laboriousness, and therefore the costliness, of the work of compilation, the difficulty of securing actual, as well as apparent, uniformity, and a consequent doubt as to the value of conclusions deduced from the figures are presumably among the causes which have defeated Miss Nightingale's scheme. Some limited portion of her object is perhaps attained by the statistical data which the administration of King's Hospital Fund demands, but even here there are possibilities of misleading comparison. There is probably no department of human inquiry in which the art of cooking statistics is unknown, and there are sceptics who have substituted 'statistics' for 'expert witnesses' in the well-known saying about classes of false statements. Miss Nightingale's scheme for Uniform Hospital Statistics seems to require for its realization a more diffused passion for statistics and a greater delicacy of statistical conscience than a voluntary and competitive system of hospitals is likely to create.

At the time she was full of hope, and, having obtained a start with medical statistics, she next pursued the subject in relation to surgical operations. Sir James Paget had been in communication with her on this point. 'We want,' he had written (Feb. 18, 1861), 'a much more exact account and a more particular record of each case. Thus in some returns we have about 40 per cent of the deaths ascribed to "exhaustion" in others, referring to the same [kind of] operations, about 3 per cent or less; the truth being that in nearly all cases of "exhaustion" there was some cause of death which more accurate inquiry would have ascertained.' Miss Nightingale (May 1, 1861) congratulated him on 'St Bartholomew's having the credit of the first Statistical Report worth having,' but the table of operations was still, she thought, most unsatisfactory. 'It would be most desirable that an uniform Table should be adopted in all Hospitals, including all the elements of age, sex, accident, habit of body, nature of operation, after-accidents, etc., etc. Could you come in to-morrow between 2 and 4, and bring your list of the causes of death after operations? It would be invaluable, coming from such an authority, for constructing a Form.' She consulted other surgeons, civil and military, and wrote a paper, with Model Forms, for the International Statistical Congress held at Berlin in September 1863. These also were included in a revised edition of *Notes on Hospitals*. The Royal College of Surgeons referred the subject to a Committee, which, however, reported adversely upon Miss Nightingale's Forms.

Before the International Congress at London in 1860 separated, Miss Nightingale addressed a letter to Lord Shaftesbury (President of the Second Section), which was read to the whole Congress, and adopted by it as a resolution. The point of it was to impress upon Governments the importance of publishing more numerous abstracts of the large amount of statistical information in their possession. She gave various instances in which useful lessons might thus be enforced upon the public mind, and cited Guizot's words: 'Valuable reports, replete with facts and suggestions drawn up by committees, inspectors, directors, and prefects, remain unknown to the public. Government ought to take care to make itself acquainted with, and promote the diffusion of all good methods, to watch our habits and institutions, there is but one instrument endowed with energy and power sufficient to secure this salutary influence—that instrument is the press.' With Miss Nightingale statistics were a passion and not merely a hobby. They did, indeed, please her, as congenial to the nature of her mind. Her correspondence with Dr Balfour and Dr Farr shows how she revelled in them. 'I have a New Year's Gift for you,' wrote Dr Farr (Jan. 1860); 'it is in the shape of Tables, as you will conjecture.' 'I am exceedingly anxious,' she replied, 'as you may suppose, to see your charming Gift, especially those Returns showing the deaths, admissions, diseases,' etc., etc. But she loved statistics, not for their own sake, but for their practical uses. It was by the statistical method that she had driven home the lessons of the Crimean hospitals. It was the study of statistics that had opened her eyes to the preventable mortality among the Army at home, and that had thus enabled her to work for the health of the British soldier. She was already engaged on similar studies in relation to India. She was in very serious, and even in bitter, earnest a 'passionate statistician.'

CENSUS RETURNS

Miss Nightingale made a valiant attempt to extend the scope of the

Census of 1861 in the interest of collecting statistical data for sanitary improvements. There were two directions in which she desired to extend the questions. One was to enumerate the numbers of sick and infirm on the Census day. For sanitary purposes it would be extremely useful to determine the proportion of sick in the different parts of the country. To those who said that it could not be done, because the people would not give the information, the answer was that it had been done in Ireland. The other point was to obtain full information about house accommodation; facts which, as would now be considered obvious, have a vital bearing on the sanitary and social conditions of the people. This point also had been covered in the Irish Census. Dr Farr entirely agreed with Miss Nightingale, but he could not persuade Sir George Lewis, the Home Secretary, to include these provisions in the Census Bill (1860). Miss Nightingale thereupon drew up a memorandum on the subject, and, through Mr Lowe (Vice-President of the Council), submitted it to the Home Secretary. Mr Lowe may have agreed with her, but he failed to persuade his colleague. 'Whenever I have power,' wrote Mr Lowe (May 9), 'you can always command me, but official omnipotence is circumscribed in the narrow limits of its own department.' Sir George Lewis replied that 'both of Miss Nightingale's points had been duly considered before the Census Bill was introduced. It was though that the question of health or sickness was too indeterminate.' 'With regard to an enumeration of houses, it was thought that this is not a proper subject to be included in a Census of population.' A very official answer! But Sir George added that he did not see how the result of such enumeration could be 'peculiarly instructive'—an avowal which he also made in the House of Commons. The cleverest of men are sometimes dense; and this remark of Sir George Lewis, added to his subsequent conduct of the War Office, earned for him, in Miss Nightingale's familiar correspondence, the sobriquet of 'The Muff.' In communicating the result of her first attempt to Dr Farr, she said, 'If you think that anything more can be done, pray say so. I'm your man.' But she had not waited to be spurred on. She had already bethought herself of a second string in the House of Lords. Lord Shaftesbury, to whom she had appealed, promised to do all he could. Lord Grey did the same, and asked her to send Dr Farr to coach him. She began to 'thank God we have a House of Lords':—

(*Miss Nightingale to Robert Lowe.*) OLD BURLINGTON ST., *May* 10 [1860]. I cannot forbear thanking you for your letter and for your exertions in our favour. Sir George Lewis's letter, *being interpreted,* means: 'Mr. Waddington does not choose to take the trouble.' It is a letter such as I have scores of in my possession, from Airey, Filder, and alas! from Lord Raglan, from Sir John Hall (the doctor) and from

Andrew Smith. It is a true 'Horse Guards' letter.

They are the very same arguments that Lord John used against the feasibility of registering the 'cause of death' in '37—which has now been the law of the land for 23 years. He was beaten in the Lords. And we are now going to fight Sir George Lewis in the Lords. And we hope to beat him too. It is mere child's play to tell us that what every man of the millions who belong to Friendly Societies does every day of his life, as to registering himself sick or well, cannot be done in the Census. It is mere childishness to tell us that it is not important to know what houses the people live in. The French Census does it. The Irish Census tell us of the great diminution of mud cabins between '41 and '51. The connection between the *health* and the *dwellings* of the population is one of the most important that exists. The 'diseases' can be obtained approximately also. In all the more important—such as small-pox, fevers, measles, heart-disease, etc.—all those which affect the *national* health, there will be very little error. (About ladies' nervous diseases there will be a great deal.) Where there *is* error in these things, the error is uniform, as is proved by the Friendly Societies; and corrects itself. . . .

The passionate statisticians were, however, hopelessly out-voted in the House of Commons. Mr Caird moved in her sense on the subject of fuller detail about house-acocommodation, and in sending her the printed notice of his amendment, said that 'his position would be greatly strengthened with the House if he could obtain Miss Nightingale's permission to quote her name in favour of the usefulness of such an inquiry.' I do not know whether she gave permission; the debate is reported very briefly in Hansard. But in any case Mr Caird's amendment was promptly negatived. As for the House of Lords, Miss Nightingale's reliance upon a better love of statistics in that assembly was cruelly falsified. The Census Bill came up late in the session, and I do not find that either Lord Grey or Lord Shaftesbury said a word upon the subject. The only critical contribution made to the debate proceeded from Lord Ellenborough, who, so far from wanting the Census Bill to include provision for more statistical data, proposed to exclude most of those that were already in. He could not for the life of him see what was the use of asking people so many questions. Here, then, Miss Nightingale was in advance of the time; in one case, by a generation, in the other, by two generations. Recent Censuses have included more particulars of the housing of the people, though still not so many as she wanted. Official statistics of the local distribution of sickness will presently be obtained, I suppose, in a different way, through the machinery of the National Health Insurance Act.

Deprived by the recalcitrance of the Home Secretary and Parliament of a fuller feast of statistics at home, Miss Nightingale turned to the Colonies and Dependencies. The Secretary for the Colonies gave her facilities for collecting much curious and instructive information;

and the Secretary of India accepted her aid in collecting and tabulating facts and figures which were the foundation of some of the most notable and beneficient of her labours. But, though she was already (1860–1) engaged in these inquiries, they belong in the main to a later period.

REFERENCE
Cook E 1913 *The Life of Florence Nightingale* vol 1 (1820–1861) (London: Macmillan) pp 428–38

Plato on Hiccoughing

This was brought to my attention in a letter by S Zak to the Editor of the *Journal of the American Medical Association* (1972) **219** 88.

Aristodemus said that it came to the turn of Aristophanes to speak; but it happened that, from repletion or some other cause, he had an hiccough which prevented him; so he turned to Eryximachus, the physician, who was reclining close beside him, and said, 'Eryximachus, it is but fair that you should cure my hiccough, or speak instead of me until it is over.'—'I will do both,' said Eryximachus, 'I will speak in your turn, and you, when your hiccough has ceased, shall speak in mine. Meanwhile, if you hold your breath some time, it will subside. If not, gargle your throat with water, and if it still continue, take something to stimulate your nostrils, and sneeze; do this once or twice, and even though it should be very violent, it will cease'—'I will follow your directions.'

[Eryximachus] '. . . for I observe your hiccough is over.' 'Yes,' said Aristophanes, 'but not before I applied the sneezing. I wonder why the harmonious construction of our body should require such noisy operations as sneezing, for it ceased the moment I sneezed.'

The Cannon Effect

Did Dmitri Shostakovich have music on the brain? An extraordinary article by a Chinese neurosurgeon in next month's *Musical Times* suggests that he had a piece of shell shrapnel lodged deep inside his brain, and that as a result each time he leaned his head to the side he

242

heard musical melodies—different each time—which he could use when composing. Moving his head back level immediately stopped the music. Dr Dajue Wang claims to have had the story from the Soviet neurosurgeon whom Shostakovich consulted, and whose x-rays allegedly located the musical fragment in the temporal horn of the left ventricle. Shostakovich was in Leningrad during the siege, but there has previously been no mention of any injury. Dr Ronald Henson, a British neurologist consulted about Wang's story, says cautiously: 'I would hesitate to affirm that it could not happen.'

REFERENCE
The Times Diary 31 May 1983

Medicine in Ancient Egypt

In Homer's *Odyssey* the Egyptian is mentioned as being unparalleled in his skill with medicine while Herodotus remarks that Egyptian schools of medicine were unrivaled in their fame and reputation. From all the known world students converged on Egypt to learn medicine, and foreign kings and princes sent to Egypt for physicians to heal them.

The origin of Egyptian superiority in this field lay in another highly developed art of those times—witchcraft. The first medicine men were priests, and as their skill was taken over by institutions of advanced learning, gradually a body of specialists developed to care for the sick in the community.

Fortunately, numerous papyri recording the medical knowledge of the ancient Egyptians have survived intact. Among these is the well-preserved Ibers papyrus, over sixty feet in length, and the most famous of such medical papyri. It is a virtual textbook of medicine and it is likely that the prescriptions recorded therein were handed down from a much earlier period, probably the Old Kingdom. Divided into 887 chapters, it embraces prescriptions for diseases of the eyes, skin, stomach, heart, arteries and bladder, as well as for gynaecological disturbances. 'Herewith begins the book of medical pharmacology for diseases of all parts of the body,' it states, and proceeds to diagnose a list of diseases and to prescribe proper treatment.

Another papyrus, that of Edwin Smith, meticulously describes surgical operations as well as the treatment of wounds in various parts of the body. It is composed of 48 chapters, each dealing with one particular case of illness, beginning with a description of the disease, followed by its symptoms, diagnosis, and treatment. The physician then gives his opinion of the case: either it is a disease he will 'treat', implying that the prospects for a cure are good; or it is a disease he will 'combat', implying that a cure is uncertain; or it is a disease he will 'not treat', implying that a cure is hopeless. This scrupulous work, obviously the product of experience and meticulous observation, is a far cry from witchcraft. In its mention of surgery, the American Egyptologist, Breasted, considers it the oldest document of its kind on record. Written during the New Kingdom the practices recorded were most likely followed in previous eras. The Hearst papyrus, too, unearthed at Dair-al-Ballas in 1899 and in poor condition, is composed of columns in which mention is made of 250 prescriptions, dating from the New Kingdom. There are many other papyri besides, preserved in museums throughout the world; they are named after their purchasers or the place of their discovery, and reveal the medical skill of the ancient Egyptian.

The earliest beginnings of medicine were probably the outcome of trial and error: a cure for a certain sickness was remembered and used at the next occurrence; and what did not work was eliminated. At this time the cause of sickness was seen to be the work of evil spirits, linking medicine to witchcraft, and most physicians were priests, who, besides prescribing medicine, used talismans and prayers to exorcize evil spirits.

It is clear from some of the medical papyri that different gods were believed to influence certain organs of the body. An appeal to the god Ra as the best cure for a scorpion sting was probably inspired by the myth of Ra extracting poison from the body of his daughter. In treating such cases the priest would call upon Ra, saying, 'O God Ra, hurry to your daughter, whom the scorpion has stung along a remote road. Her screams pierce the skies. The poison runs beneath her skin, spreading throughout her body. She licks the wounded spot like a cat.' Ra would reply, 'Don't be scared. Don't be scared, my daughter, for here I stand behind you.'

The medical profession gradually developed a vocational creed which was passed down from one generation to another, and eventually formed the basis of the Hippocratic oath. Centres for the teaching of medicine were also established. The author of the Ibers papyrus writes, 'I graduated from the University of Heliopolis, together with the princes of the great household, the masters of protection and the rulers of eternity.' That there were such schools of medicine in Heliopolis, Sais, and Memphis is certain.

One of the most famous of ancient physicians was Imhotep, who practiced during the reign of King Zoser in the 28th century BC. After his death he was elevated to godhood by the ancient Egyptians, and the Greeks knew him as Asclepius, the god of healing.

Herodotus pointed out that Egyptian medicine was divided into various fields, each of which had its specialists, but there were also special physicians for the populace, the army, and the royal court. One group of doctors specialized in the use of herbs and the recital of prayers, while another specialized in the use of bandages.

Treatment was divided accordingly into that of internal disorders and that of external disorders, the latter also included surgery, and required experience, skill, and accurate observation. Treatment of internal disorders called for a knowledge of medicine and witchcraft.

One medical papyrus describes catarrh and its treatment. A talisman, which was often read after administering the medicine, gives a precise description of the symptoms of the catarrh:

> Get away catarrh, son of catarrh, which breaks the bones, crushes the skull, pierces the brain, and affects the seven apertures of the head. I have brought a medicine to combat you.

The Ibers papyrus reveals a knowledge of the function of veins and arteries.

It also touched upon gynaecology, prescribed a method to judge a woman's fertility, as well as the quality of mother's milk by its odour.

Surgery is described in the Edwin Smith papyrus, which says specialists in this field were priests devoted to the god Sikhoset, who conducted minor operations such as circumcision and the opening of abscesses. They could differentiate between fractures and dislocations of the bones and they knew how to make splints. Wounds were bandaged after an application of fresh meat, honey, or fat.

After the diagnosis the appropriate medicine was selected from an apparently large number of available preparations, some of which were fast-working and others not, some prescribed for summer and others for winter. If the patient was an adolescent or an adult, medicine was given in the form of pills, but if the patient was still a child, it was mixed with the mother's milk.

I might mention here that in the margins of every medical papyrus, beside the prescriptions, there are such notations as 'good', 'useful', or 'good, I saw it administered and prepared it myself.'

Some of the medicines used, such as the eye medicine, were imported from the city of Jabail on the Phoenician coast. Other medicines were known as cure-alls, called repellents of death, and considered the concoctions of Ra, who had invented them for use against his own senility. Such medicine, made of honey, wax, and fourteen kinds of herbs, was applied in the form of a plaster to the painful area.

Medicine to be taken orally came in the form of pills or syrups, and that to be applied externally was made into ointments or plasters. The prescription indicated whether the medicine was to be mixed, ground, or pounded.

Perhaps the skill of the ancient Egyptians in medicine explains their expertise at mummification, the art of preserving the body from decay. It is uncertain exactly when Egyptians began to practice mummification, which ended with the spread of Christianity, but we know that in prehistoric times the dead were buried in relatively shallow pits after being first wrapped in mats, skins, flax, or the like. The dryness of the climate and the heat of the sun dehydrated the body and preserved it as long as it remained dry. Because of the difference in weather conditions, mummifying through dehydration could be successfully carried out in Upper Egypt but not in the delta.

The first Egyptians to note the effects of dehydration must have been greatly astonished to discover, as they went into the desert to bury the dead, that the body of a grandfather or great-grandfather was still so well preserved. It was perhaps this kind of experience that led the early Egyptians to a belief in an afterlife and resurrection. To the ancients the body was like a box containing various substances that could exist eternally, but only on condition that the body was preserved. It was also for this reason that tombs were provided with food and water at the time of burial.

The first reliable evidence of mummification, according to the famous chemist Lucas, dates from the beginning of the Fourth Dynasty. Lucas found, through examining the intestines of Queen Hetub Hars, mother of King Cheops, builder of the Great Pyramid of Giza, that the embalming fluid was composed of natron, sodium sulphate, and sodium chloride.

The process of dehydration of the body was done in two ways: by the sun or by fire; or by the use of absorbent materials. Dehydration of the body through the action of the sun is slow, since 75 per cent of body weight is water. If the body is wrapped in skin, mat, or flax and buried in a dry place exposed to the sun, it loses moisture through the absorbing action of the sand. This process was found accidentally in prehistoric times but later became one of two ways of mummification, though it was not suited for general use.

Herodotus left us a description of embalmment in which he says that the specialists of this trade made available to the family of the deceased three wooden models of embalmment at three different prices. The embalming process, which greatly impressed Herodotus, called for the extraction of most of the brain through the nostrils by means of an iron hook and medical dissolvents. The abdomen was cut to remove the intestines, and body cavity washed out with date wine

246

mixed with spices, later to be filled with incense. The incision was then sewn up and the body placed in natron for seventy days, after which it was washed once again and wrapped with flax saturated in glue. This was then handed over to the family, who would encase it in a coffin to be placed in a tomb.

Herodotus also describes a second, cheaper method, in which the body was injected with rice oil through the anus. It was then placed in natron for seventy days, during which time the rice oil leaked out with the dissolved intestines.

The third method mentioned by Herodotus, one used by the poor, called for cleaning out the body with a laxative solution, then placing it seventy days in natron.

Diodorus Siculus, on the other hand, who presumably knew the words of Herodotus, mentions only one method of embalmment, similar to the first one, where the abdomen was cut to remove the intestines, heart, and kidneys, then washed with date wine mixed with spices and perfumed with incense.

In considering these accounts we must keep in mind that both Herodotus and Diodorus were describing embalming as practiced at a late stage in Egyptian history. Herodotus visited Egypt between 448 and 445 BC, Diodorus in 59 BC. In Lucas's opinion, Herodotus is generally more accurate in his description, although the details of his account would probably vary from those of earlier ages. The period during which the body was placed in natron, in particular, has been an object of debate among scholars.

REFERENCE
Abdel-Kader H 1982 *Life in Ancient Egypt* 2nd edn (Cairo: Al Ahram Commercial Press) 98–105

Anecdote of Aesclepiades of Prusa

Aesclepiades was a Greek physician who practised in Rome during the first century BC. So confident was he of his own medical competence that he maintained he would no longer claim the title of physician should he ever become ill. Subsequently he had the good taste to die, while still in the bloom of health, by plunging down a staircase. His reputation survived his fatal fall!

The First Whole-Body X-Ray

This radiograph was taken in 1896 in New York and published in the *Archives of the Roentgen Ray*, London. The exposure lasted 30 minutes. Clothing and jewellery which can be seen include: a hatpin, necklace, rings, bracelet, high buttoned boots with a buckle, nail heel shoes and a whalebone corset.

(Copyright.)
ENTIRE ADULT BODY AT ONE EXPOSURE.
(By WILLIAM J. MORTON, M.D., N.Y.)
PLATE XXX. (b).

Meo Hill Tribe Herb Doctor in Northern Thailand

On a visit to Thailand in 1985 I saw the villag of the Meo Tribe, near the Golden Triangle, in the far north of Thailand beyond Chiangmai and beyond the temple of Doi Suthep at 1056 metres.

A village market was present with all the usual wood carvings, carpets and knick-knacks, but in addition there was the stall of the village 'herb doctor'. Most remedies cost some 20 Bahts (£0.75), such as:

> *Tiger strength*
>> for backache
>
> *The bandit has been killed from the sky*
>> for intestinal cancer and for haemorroids
>
> *God given*
>> for arthritis and for muscle pain
>
> *Cardamom*
>> for heart disease, for dizziness and for vertigo
>
> *Bitter root*
>> for diabetes, for nephritis and for cystitis

The bandit has been killed from the sky (for intestinal cancer).

God given (for arthritis and muscle pain).

Cardamom (for heart disease, dizziness and vertigo).

Erecting (for impotence).

However, the most interesting hard sell, via an interpreter, came when the herb doctor tried to persuade me to buy a tiger's penis for 1500 Baht (£50). This medicinal item was baked in honey and was used by dissolving it in a jar of locally brewed alcohol, and then 15 ml was prescribed orally each day. One tiger's penis was said to last a year and was supposed to be the best aphrodisiac anywhere in the world.

The herb doctor.

I then had to explain that I was not a rich American, to which the herb doctor replied with a statement of why 1500 Baht was a reasonable price. 'First, you have to catch your tiger, and then there is only one penis per tiger, so it has to be 1500 Baht.'

Finally, the herb doctor must have felt sorry for me, or else the doctor friend interpreter gave him instructions, but whatever the reason, I was presented with the 20 Baht version of an aphrodisiac, which has the name Erecting.

Anatomical Comparisons by Rabelais

Lungs like a fur-lined hood
Heart like a chasuble
Mediastinum like forceps
Arteries like a watchman's cloak
Diaphragm like a cockaded cap
Liver like a double axe
Veins like canvas window blinds

Jail Fever in Newgate

In the early part of the eighteenth century, for every person hanged at Tyburn, four would die of jail fever in Newgate prison before they could be hanged. Jail fever was the result of bad sanitation and over-crowding and it was not limited to London; for example in 1577 at an assize in Oxford, some 300 persons died.

At Newgate, the epidemic also extended to the adjoining Sessions House and in 1750 the fever struck down more than 60 people, including jurymen, barristers, the Lord Mayor of London, Under Sheriff and also a former Lord Mayor. As a result, the jail had to be virtually sterilised and was to this end washed down with vinegar. Similarly, prisoners were washed down with vinegar before they were brought to trial, and from this time judges carried with them, and had on the bench, a nosegay of flowers to ward off the prison smells.

Thus from a 1772 document:

> To keep out the foul air while in court, candied orange peel or lemon peel, preserved gingers, and garlic if not disagreeable, cardamon, carraway, or other confits, may be very useful, and should the mouth

be clammed, dry raisins, currants, or lemon drops, will cool, and quench thirst, which, should it increase, may be assuaged by small draughts of old hock and water, or small punch. Smelling to good wine vinegar during the trials, will not only refresh, but revive, more agreeably and cool, than the use of spirituous waters distilled from lavender or rosemary, and more than any other scents.

and

To guard the seat of justice from the approaches of infection, it will certainly be most prudent to fumigate and steam the place, by means of large braziers, pans or coppers, put in the day before the sessions are to commence, and during that day to burn in them charcoal, with tobacco stalks, and dried aromatic herbs in winter, as mint, rosemary, southern-wood etc., bruised juniper berries may also be burnt; and on a hot iron shovel may be put wet gunpowder, and frankincense, but particularly the steams of boiling hot vinegar should be conveyed to all parts of the building. The next morning about an hour or two before the court meet, the braziers should be filled with coke cinders, as used by maltsters instead of charcoal, and after they shall have burned awhile, the ventilator should let in fresh air, and the floor should be sprinkled with cold vinegar of the sharpest sort. At the time of opening the court, the air-holes, made close to the ground, about a foot square, should be set open and the wooden flaps hooked up.

THE OLD SESSIONS HOUSE IN THE OLD BAILEY IN 1750.

The old Sessions House in the Old Bailey, 1750. (Courtesy Mansell Collection.)

One suggestion for improving Newgate conditions was to con-struct a windmill on the roof of the gatehouse which it was hoped

252

would draw off the poisonous air. The medical theory was that stale air putrifies and that this in turn dissolves the blood and humours of the human body to set up further putrefaction which would ultimately dissolve the human body itself! Several workmen engaged in the windmill exercise became ill from the smell and this mirrored what happened two years earlier for a similar windmill at London's Bridewell prison. Then, workmen had refused to carry out the work unless they were given tobacco and drink as precautionary measures. Surprisingly, they stayed immune, but some carpenters who worked with them and did not insist on the same conditions got jail fever, and two of them died.

REFERENCES

Anon 1772 *Directions to Prevent the Contagion of the Jail—Distemper Commonly Called Jail-Fever* (London)

Rumblelow D 1982 *The Triple Tree: Newgate, Tyburn and Old Bailey* (London: Harrap)

Diderot on Doctors

The best doctor is the one you run for and cannot find.

John Hunter on Operations

Never perform an operation on another person which, under similar circumstances, you would not have performed on yourself.

On Alcoholism

An alcoholic is someone you do not like who drinks as much as you.

Witch from Brittany

Carved wood figure of a witch. Breton workmanship from Treanton Morlaix. The witch is using a pestle and mortar and has a cat on her shoulder. (Courtesy Wellcome Institute Library, London.)

Moscow Weddings

When young Muscovites get married, many of them follow a pattern which leaves parents, aunts and uncles at home getting an enormous party ready, whilst the happy couple tour the major sites of Moscow. These include the grave of the unknown warrior in the Alexandrovsky Gardens by the Kremlin Wall, the Lenin Hills below the University of Moscow (where photographs are taken with a panoramic view of Moscow in the background), and the large black wooden crosses a few kilometres from the airport, which mark the nearest point to Moscow reached by Hitler's army in what is termed, in the USSR, The Great Patriotic War (World War II). One quaint custom often observed is for the wedding car to have a Russian doll or a Russian teddy bear attached to the radiator grille. I was told on good authority that this would ensure either a girl baby (for those with a doll) or a boy baby (for those with a bear). Whenever I have seen a group of wedding cars, dolls always seem to outnumber bears in a ratio of 10:1. However, since this ratio bears no relation to the actual Russian population statistics, this predictive technique is a failure!

On Filling in Life Insurance Forms

When the death penalty was still in force in the United Kingdom, an Englishman and an American were exchanging experiences on the problem of completing life insurance forms when, as in both their cases, their fathers were found guilty of murder and the ultimate sentence was passed on them. The American's solution was to write that his father met with an accident when he was in the Chair of Applied Electricity, whereas the Englishman's solution was to write that his father died when the platform gave way at a public event.

255

Saint Pantaleon

Patron saint of physicians in the Eastern Church and a patron saint of consumption. From a fourteenth-century Greek manuscript in the Bibliothèque Nationale, Paris. (Courtesy Wellcome Institute Library, London.)

On How to Start a Speech in the Apothecaries Hall

In a dinner in 1988 in the Apothecaries Hall in the City of London, the Master of one of the City Livery Companies began his speech with the following information. 'A recent survey of city businessmen gathered together for a meeting in a room at any time yielded the following statistic. 66% are thinking about sex. I therefore hope that two-thirds of you are enjoying yourselves. . . .'

256

On Getting Matters into Perspective

Two Canadian backpackers encountered a grizzly bear on their trek through the woods. Immediately one of them removed his pack, and as quickly as possible put on his running shoes. The other stood in amazement and said 'That is no good, the grizzly can run a lot faster than you.' 'Ah' said his friend, 'but I don't have to run faster than the bear, I only have to run faster than you.'

A Moralistic Story About Two Peasants, a Bird and a Cow

In the bitter cold of winter, in a small village during a howling gale and with darkness falling, a peasant is wandering home to his meagre village. Suddenly he stops as he sees a small game bird on the ground, nearly dead from cold and privation. The peasant picks up the bird and warms it. The bird soon recovers and the peasant wonders what to do next. At that moment a herd of cattle come by and one of them drops a large dollop right in front of him. Realising that if he puts the bird in the steaming cow's dollop, the bird will stay warm until morning and then be able to fly away, he does this and then goes home. But a second peasant comes along after the first one has gone and hears the bird chirping happily to itself in the steaming mess. This peasant seizes the bird, breaks its neck and takes it home for supper.

This story has three morals:

1 Do not believe that everybody who drops you in the shit is your enemy.
2 Do not believe that everybody who gets you out of the shit is your friend.
3 Whenever you *are* in the shit keep quiet about it.

International Definitions of Heaven and Hell

Heaven: Italian cooks, English police, a French mistress, German car mechanics and the Swiss undertaking any necessary organising
Hell: English cooks, German police, a Swiss mistress, French car mechanics and the Italians doing the organising

These definitions were told by a Russian national working at the World Health Organisation in Geneva, as the WHO in-joke of 1987. It was noticeable that no Russian attributes figured in the anecdote!

The Frog

The humble frog has found its way into medical applications, such as in 1896, one year after the discovery of X-rays, when it was used as a test object, one of the earliest in diagnostic radiology, to demonstrate the 'new light'.

Earlier than Röntgen's discovery of X-rays, its name was taken to describe a thermometer, invented around 1650 in Florence. The Frog Thermometer was a strange contraption shaped like a large hollow glass frog. It was filled half-way with water containing glass beads of different colours according to their specific gravity. Fixation to someone's body was by means of ribbons so that the belly of the frog would be in contact with the skin. The water would warm up and become lighter in proportion, and the glass beads would rearrange themselves according to their own specific gravity or colour. From their position and colour, the temperature was estimated.

The frog is still used in this context today. In a *New Scientist* editorial dwelling on the world's slow perception of the extent and importance of AIDS, deforestation, desertification, the greenhouse

258

effect and the hole in the ozone layer, the following was written. 'If you take a frog from its pond and put it in a pan of hot water, it will jump out. If you put it in a pan of cold water and heat it slowly on the stove, the frog will sit there until it boils to death. The frog's senses are equipped to measure only large differences in temperature, not gradual ones. It has evolved that way because it normally has no need to measure gradual changes in temperature. Today, the human race has a lot in common with the frog in the pot'.

REFERENCES
Mould R F 1985 *A History of X-rays and Radium* (Sutton: IPC Business Press)
New Scientist 17 June 1989
Sterpellone L 1988 *Instruments for Health* (Milan: Farmitalia Carlo Erba)

Sales Opportunities!

The following is a newspaper cutting of May 1982 which appeared with the caption 'Nuns Arrested'. It was contributed by Mr Tony O'Connor.

When a group of nuns spent over £2 million on a new convent in northern Belgium, officials launched an investigation into how the funds were raised. Now the Mother Superior and a senior nun are under arrest, charged with defrauding the Health Service of £7 million. It is alleged they encouraged doctors to sign blank treatment forms, then got other sisters to claim payment for health work never carried out.

Bulgarian Proverb

Nature, time and patience are the three great physicians.

Irish Proverb

Death is the poor man's best physician.

A Medical Demon From Angkor Wat

Ravana, King of the Rakshas, a demon to whom were attributed several medical works. Bas-relief from Angkor Wat. (Courtesy Wellcome Institute Library, London.)

Confusion

Contributed by a sales manager who wishes to remain nameless!

'I fully realise that I have not succeeded in answering all of your questions. . . . Indeed, I feel I have not answered any of them completely. The answers I have found only serve to raise a whole new set of questions, which only lead to more problems, some of which we weren't even aware were problems. To sum it all up . . . in some ways I feel we are as confused as ever, but I believe we are confused on a higher level, and about more important things.'

Index

Abortions, 182
Acapulco, 164
Adults, 126
Afghanistan, 133
Agate, 47
Agrippina (16–59 AD), 14
Alcohol, 68, 99–101, 106, 164, 177, 180, 181, 219, 253, 257
Alcoholism, 253
Alexander the Great (356–323 BC), 14, 20–3
Alligator, 82
Amber, 47
Ambulance, 133
America, *see* USA
American giant, 24, 26
Amethyst, 47
Amputation, 44, 51, 217
Anaemia, 187
Anaesthetics, 40, 161, 228–33
Anatomy, 27–31, 109, 125, 176, 202, 203, 223, 245, 251
Angkor Wat, 260
Annointing, 156
Anorexia nervosa, 93
Antivisectionist, 107
Ants, 50
Aphrodisiac, 250
Apothecary, 166
Arab medicine, 87
Archives of Clinical Skiagraphy, 7
Archives of the Roentgen Ray, 7
Arm, 117
Arthritis, 40, 259
Asclepiades (140–24 BC), 112, 247
Asklepios, 106, 126, 174
Aspel, Michael, 42
Assyria, 50, 106
Asthma, 69, 70
Astrology, 203
Astronomy, 102, 103
Australia, 42, 111, 153, 225
Austria, 14, 175, 179
Authors, 59, 84
Autographs, 141

Babylonian medicine, 41, 50, 68, 106, 130
Backache, 249
Bahamas, 181
Balkan medicine, 152
Barber–Surgeons, 82, 198
Barnum's prize ladies, 34
Bathtub elixir, 219
Belgium, 166, 259
The Bible, 88
Biddenden maids, 35
Billings, John Shaw (1838–1913), 59
Biology, 107
Bismarck, Otto von (1815–1898), 178
Bladder, bladder stone, 48, 151
Blood letting, 83, 84
Blue men, 73–81
Bogorov vodka, 181
Bohemia, 180
Bombs, 120
Bookmakers, 177
Brain, 48, 118, 178
Brazil, 188
Bread buttering, 102–5
Breast cancer, 109
Brideshead Revisited, TV series, 19
Broken arm, 117
Bronchitis, 45, 69
Buck-passing machine, 128–9
Bullets, 59, 117
Bull fighting, 164
Burial, 222
Butler, Samuel (1835–1902), 176
Byron, Lord (1788–1824), 214–18

Caesarean section, 58
Cairo, 98
Cambodia, 260
Camel ambulance, 133
Canada, 97, 117, 165, 257
Cancer, 58, 109, 193, 249
Capgras syndrome, 220
Carbolic smoke ball, 69
Catarrh, 245

Cavities, 127
Census returns, 239
Chamfort, Nicholas (1741–1794) 125
Champagne, 49
Chang–Eng Bunker, Siamese
    twins, 5
Charms, 152, 153, 154
Chernobyl accident, 180–5
Chiangmai, 249
Childbirth, 54, 58, 60, 196, 212–14,
    255
Childhood, 167–72
China, 31, 44, 84, 163, 164, 242
Chiropody, 40, 185, 186
Churchill, Sir Winston (1874–1965),
    96, 141
Cigarettes, 81
Cigars, 45
Ciliary muscles, 108
Claudius (10 BC–54 AD), Emperor
    of Rome, 149
Clavicle, 185, 186
Clinical trials, 88
Cobalt-60 radiotherapy machine, 17
Cockneys, 176, 202–3
Coffin, 26
Computers, 4
Confucius (551–479 BC), 44
Conan Doyle, Sir Arthur
    (1859–1930), *see also* Sherlock
    Holmes, 190–5
Confusion, 260
Consumption, 70
Contraception, 221
Copernicus, Nicholas (1473–1543),
    102–5
Coral, 47
Cows, 33, 99, 162, 257
Cow pearl jam, 98
Cramps, 50
Crimean War hospitals
    (1854–1856), 205–12, 234
Cripples, 57
Crisps, 201
Croup, 69
Cuba, 14, 188, 224
Cures, 50, 68, 69, 70
Cystitis, 249

Deafness, 225
Death, *see* Last words
De Medicina (30 AD), 4
Demosthenes (382–322 BC), 23
Denmark, 14
Dental identification, 14
Dentist, *see* Teeth, Toothache,
    Surgeon–Dentist
Dermatology, 40
Descartes, René (1596–1650), 24
Diabetes, 249
Diagnosis, 43, 48, 86, 109, 163, 186,
    243–7
Diamond, 45
Dickens, Charles (1812–1870), 141
Diderot, Denis (1713–1784), 253
Diet, 160, 201
Digitalis, 34
Dislocation of the neck, 37
Dissection, 28, 34, 35
Diuretic, 106
Divorce, 123
Drugs and drug prescriptions, 48,
    125
Duels, 178
Dwarfs and giants, 24–7
Dying words, *see* Last words

Earache, 185, 186
East India Company, 139
Easter Sunday, 35
Economics, 84
Egypt, 14–23, 98, 185–7, 243
Egyptian medicine, 185–7, 243–7
Egyptology, *see* Mummies
Electric chair, 255
Epilepsy, 108, 177
Estonia, 219
Eustachian tube, 107
Evil spirits, stuffed alligator, 82
Examinations, 107
Experiment with rats, 52
Experiment with mice, 181
Explosives, 120, 153
Eyes, 48, 58, 101, 108
Eye operation, 41

Falling downstairs, 116, 247
Falling off a ladder, 120
False teeth, 115
Famine, 185
Fees, 32, 39, 40, 41, 43, 163
Fever, 112, 223, 224, 251–3
Fibonacci (1175–1230), 147
Finger reckoning, 147
Fire damage, 33
Floral tributes, 164
Florence, University, Wax
    Museum, 27–31
Forceps, 62, 196
Foreheads, 148–52
Foxgloves, 34
France, 1, 14, 86, 119, 120, 175, 196,
    204, 220, 221, 225, 254
Franco-Prussian war (1870–1871),
    1, 225
Frogs, 258

Gallstones, 164
Gem stones, 45–8
Generals, 50
George VI (1895–1952), 176
Gerasimov, Professor Mikhail
    (1907–1970), 9–14
Germany, 102, 178, 221
Giants and dwarfs, 24–7
Gilmore, James (1885–1963), 41
Gin, 99–101, 257
God, 42
Golden Triangle, 249
Gonorrhea, 44, 58, 203
Gorky Park, novel, 9
Graphology, 135–47
Gravestone inscription, 51
Greece, 14–23, 39, 50, 86, 106, 126,
    182, 247
Grizzly bear, 257
Guinness, 164, 166
Guthrie, George James
    (1795–1856), 37–9
Gynaecology, 163

Haemorrhoids, 37, 110
Hair, 134

Handwriting, *see also* Graphology,
    123, 141, 145
Hangover, 68
Hay fever, 69
Headache, 69
Heart failure, 40, 249
Heaven and Hell, 258
Henry VIII (1509–1547), 48, 149
Herb doctor, 250
Hernia, 44
Hiccoughs, 242
Hindu medicine, 46, 50
Hippocrates (460–357 BC), 37, 64,
    65, 106
Hogarth, William (1697–1764),
    99–101
Holland, *see* Netherlands
Homer (*c.* 850 BC), 106, 243
Horse doctor, 59
Human race, 259
Hungary, 180
Hunter, John (1728–1793), 24–7, 253

Identikit and photofit techniques,
    13
Immortality, 163
Impotence, 162, 250
Incantation, 106
India, 46
Infertility, 56
Insurance forms, 255
Intestines, 48, 58, 249
Ireland, 24, 58, 105, 162, 201
Irish giant, 25–6
Italy, *including* Rome, 4, 27–31, 39,
    49, 60–8, 85, 112, 148, 173,
    247
Ivan the Terrible (1530–1584), 9

Jade, 48
Jail fever, 251–3
Jam, 98
Jenner, Edward (1749–1823), 107,
    224
Jewish medicine, 152

Khan el Khalili bazaar, 98
Khnum-Nakht (12th Dynasty),
    14–17

Kidneys, 48, 249
Koko, 134
Kuwait, 163

Laboratory of Plastic
    Reconstruction, Moscow,
    9–14
Lancashire prodigy (1838), 8
Lapis lazuli, 47
La Specola, Wax Museum of
    Florence, 27–31
Last words, 49, 123
Law student, 120
Legs, 51, 117, 185, 186
Lepers, 57
Life insurance forms, 255
Limb setting, 85
Linear accelerator for radiotherapy,
    17
Lisbon, 1
Liverpool, 81, 139
Lobotomy, 220
London cockneys, *see* Cockneys
Louis XIV (1643–1715), 28
Louis XVI (1774–1792), 176
Lung, removal, 41
Lung pills, 70
Luther, Martin (1483–1546), 31
Luxembourg, 221

Macedonia, 14–23
Magic, 43, 249–51
Malingering, 88–97
Malpractice, 119
Malungay plant, 187
Manchester University, 14–23
Manioc root, 187–90
Manipulation, 51
Mascagni, Paolo (1755–1815), 27, 29
Mathematics, 31, 147
Maugham, Somerset (1874–1965), 59
Medical
    demon, 260
    fees, *see* Fees
    journals, 59
    papyri, 185–187, 243
    students, 34, 111, 112, 176

Medici, 28, 197
Medicine man, Australia, 43
Medico-legal matters, 116–23
Mesmer, Anton (1734–1815), 174–6
Mesmerism, 174–6, 233
Metoposcopy, 148–52
Mexico, 164
Mice, 181, 204
Milk transfusion, 97
Mind, 24
Mistakes in surgery, 41, 119
Modelling with plaster of Paris and
    alginate, 17
Modelling with wax, 27–31
Mole's feet, 154
Monologues, 130–3, 155–6
Monsters, bicephalic and
    parasitic, 8, 33
Montgomery, Lord (1887–1976), 174
Morton, William (1820–1868),
    228–33
Moscow weddings, 254, 255
Moslem medicine, 46, 87
Mother's ruin, 99
Mummies, Egyptian, 14–23, 246
Munchausen's syndrome, 93, 95,
    96
Murder, 4, 12, 118, 119, 161, 177,
    255

Naevus, 151
Nansen, Fridtjof (1861–1930), 112
Napoleon Bonaparte (1769–1821), 39
Napoleon III (1808–1873), 1
National Health Service, 48, 259
National registration numbers in
    Sweden, 4
Nebuchadnezzar, 88
Nekht-Ankh (12th Dynasty),
    14–17
Nelson, Lord (1758–1805), 139–47,
    178
Neolithic man, 10
Nestor, 67
Netherlands, 33, 71, 99, 200
Neuralgia, 69
New York, 73–81, 98
Newgate jail, 251

Nightingale, *Florence* (1820–1910), 205–12, 233–42
Nightingale, two-headed, 33
Nightmares, 153
Norway, 14, 112
Nosebleeds, 110
Nuclear accidents, *see* Chernobyl accident
Nuclear leak, 164
Nuns, 259
Nurses and nursing, *see also* Florence Nightingale, 1
Nursing mothers, 57

Obesity, 34, 98
Obstetrics, *see* Childbirth
Odontology, Forensic departments, 14
Onions, 106
Opal, 47
Opium, 130–3
'Orphan Annie' eyes, 101
Orris root, 152
Oruncha, magic healing crystal, 42–3
Owen, John (1560–1622), 42
Oysters, 107
Oyster/Carlisle, Sir Anthony (1768–1840), 227

Palmerston, Lord (1784–1865), 123
Panama, 83
Paracelsus (1493–1541), 46, 47
Parotid, 193
Patients, 1, 39, 177
Peasants, 257
Peninsular War (1808–1814), 38, 39
Persia, 125, 179
Personality, 160
Pestäule, Vienna, 180
Pharmacy and pharmacists, 48, 166, 200, 254
Philip II of Macedon (died 336 BC), 14, 20–3
Philip III Arrhidaeus (died 317 BC), 20
Phillipines, 187
Philosophy, 125

Physicians, 5, 32, 36, 39, 43, 86, 124, 253
Pig's feet, 153
Pigtail, 31, 32, 130–3
Plague, 104, 151, 179, 223
Plato (429–347 BC), 242
Pliny (23–79 AD), 39
Poaching, 51
Poison, 151, 244
Poland, 152
Polar expeditions, 112
Poliomyelitis, 185, 186
Political prisoners, 160
Pompeii and Herculaneum, 60–8
Pope, Alexander (1688–1744), 142
Pope Clement VII (1478–1534), 46
Portugal, 1
Post mortem, 164
Postal franking before introduction of stamps, 142
Pregnancy, 37, 108, 162, 163
Prince Charles' wedding, 159
Prison, 115, 162, 165, 251
Private patients, 39
Proctologists, 164
Proverbs,
    Bulgarian, 259
    French, 86
    Irish, 105, 259
    Spanish, 32
Public House signs, 162

Quacks, 44, 71–3, 173, 190

Rabelais, Francois (1494–1553), 251
Rabbits, 153
Radiation protection, 124
Radiotherapy, 17
Radium, 115
Rats, 52
Reconstruction of a face, 9–14
The Red Cross, 1–3
Red Indian medicine, 83
Rejecting a manuscript, 84
Revolvers, 59
Reynolds, Sir Joshua (1723–1792), 24
Rheumatism, 154
Rhubarb, 127

Richelieu, Duc de (1585–1642), 123
Robot, 220
Roman surgeons, 4
Rome, see Italy
Royal College of Surgeons, 24, 37
Rudaki, Tadjik poet (died 10th
    Century), 13
Ruptures, 36
Russia, see USSR

Saints,
    Anthony's Fire, 55
    Eufrasia of Pisa, 37
    George and the dragon, 56
    Hildegard, 46
    in Names of hospitals, 53–8
    Pantaleon, 256
Salamanca, battle of, 39
Salerno, Roger of (13th Century), 85
Saracens, 88
Sausages, 178
Scorpion sting, 244
Sewage, 107
Sex and statistics, 256
Sex change operations, 163
Sherlock Holmes and Doctor Watson,
    91, 113–14
Shostacovich, Dmitri (born 1906),
    242
Shrewsbury, Earl of (1373–1453),
    204
Siamese twins, 5–8
Sicilian dwarf, 24, 27
Sicily, 24, 60, 88
Sin, 31
Sing Sing prison, 115
Skeletons, 25
Slang, 202–3
Smallpox, 107, 224
Snoring, 69, 165
Space technology, 201
Spain, 32, 38, 39, 46, 114, 164
Specialists, 124
Speech, 178, 256
Spleen, 48
Statistics, 52, 59, 165, 233–42, 256
St Louis, USA, 43
Stomach pains, 109, 114

Students, see Medical students
Suffragettes, 160
Suicide, 39, 155–6, 161, 162, 177,
    221
Surgeon's house in Pompeii, 66
Surgeon–Dentist, 179
Surgery and surgeons, 4, 25, 36,
    37–9, 41, 50, 60–8, 82, 176,
    179, 190–5, 232, 253
Surgical instruments, 63
Susini, Clemente (1754–1805), 27, 28
Swallowing, 114, 115
Sweden, 4
Switzerland, 176, 258
Symptoms, 37
Syndromes, 220
Syphilis, 44, 58, 203
Syria, 174

Talavera, battle of, 39
Tattoos, 158, 159
Teeth, 44, 49, 52, 53, 152, 179, 190
Terrorism (1896), 120
Thailand, 249–51
Theology, 31
Thermometers, 177, 258
Thessaloniki University, 20
Thomas, Sir Clement Price
    (1894–1973), 176
Tiger's penis, 250
Tombstones, 49, 86
Toothache, 49, 58
Toronto, 97, 165
Toulouse, battle of, 39
Trafalgar, battle of, 141
Transfusion, milk, 97
Transport requests to clinic, 40
Trepanning, 64, 108
Trichinosis, 178
Trojan War, 106
Trusses, 36
Tuberculosis, 108
Turkey, 50, 92
Turquoise, 47
Twins, 5–8, 178

Uganda, 58
Undertaker, 26

Urine, 71–3
Urologists, 164
USA, 24, 43, 51, 69, 73–81, 83, 115,
    119, 120, 127, 157, 164, 201,
    220, 228, 255
USSR, 9–14, 180–5, 219, 225, 242,
    254, 258
Uterus, 108

Vaccination, 225
Varicose veins, 126
Vergina, Macedonia, 20
Vertigo, 249
Vets, 33
Vices, 177
Vimeiro, battle of, 38
Virchow, Rudolf (1821–1902), 178
Vodka, 180, 181
Voltaire, Francoise-Marie Arouet
    (1694–1778), 5

Washington, George (1732–1799), 127
Water doctor, 71–3
Waterloo, battle of, 39, 144
Wax Museum of Florence, 27–31
Wellington, Duke of (1769–1852),
    38–9, 139–47
Westminster Hospital, 38, 176, 226
Whooping cough, 69

Wife murder, 118
Wilde, Oscar (1854–1900), 49
Wilson, Edward Bidwell
    (1879–1964), 52
Wine, medicinal uses, 45, 106
Witch, 254
Wolf's tooth, 153
Wordsworth, William (1770–1850),
    93
World Health Organisation, 258
Wound closure, 50, 114

X-rays, 114–23, 124, 220, 258
X-ray pictures, skiagrams,
    radiographs,
    double monster (1896), 7
    false teeth swallowed (1902), 115
    bullet in the brain (1896), 118
    whole body (1896), 248

Yellow fever, 224
Yorkshire water doctor, 71–3

Zaire, 187
Zips, 114
Zummo (Zumbo), Gaetano Guilio
    (1665–1701), 28, 29